ICF

ICF

A Hands-on Approach for Clinicians and Families

Edited by Olaf Kraus de Camargo, Liane Simon,
Gabriel M Ronen and Peter L Rosenbaum

2019
Mac Keith Press

Managing Director: Ann-Marie Halligan
Project Management: Riverside Publishing Solutions Ltd

First published in this edition in 2019 by Mac Keith Press
2nd Floor, Rankin Building, 139–143 Bermondsey Street, London, SE1 3UW

British Library Cataloguing-in-Publication data
A catalogue record for this book is available from the British Library

Cover design: Hannah Rogers
Cover illustration: Navita Dyal
Icons on front cover made by Freepik, Skyclick and Prosymbols from www.flaticon.com

ISBN: 978-1-911612-04-9

Typeset by Riverside Publishing Solutions Ltd

Printed by Hobbs the Printers Ltd, Totton, Hampshire, UK

Contents

SECTION C

Appendix 6: The ICF code sets for children and youth are available to download online at
http://www.mackeith.co.uk/shop/icf-a-hands-on-approach-for-clinicians-and-families/

Author Appointments

Jennifer Johannesen
Parent and Bioethicist, Toronto, Canada

Olaf Kraus de Camargo
Associate Professor, Department of Paediatrics, McMaster University; Scientist, CanChild Centre for Childhood Disability Research, McMaster University; Developmental Paediatrician, Ron Joyce Children's Health Centre of McMaster Children's Hospital, Hamilton, Ontario, Canada

Jaclyn Pederson
Senior Director of Programs and Strategic Initiatives, Feeding Matters, Phoenix, AZ, USA

Gabriel M Ronen
Professor of Paediatrics (Paediatric Neurology), McMaster University and McMaster Children's Hospital, Hamilton, Ontario, Canada

Peter L Rosenbaum
Professor of Paediatrics, McMaster University; Co-founder, CanChild Centre for Childhood Disability Research, McMaster University, Hamilton, Ontario, Canada

Liane Simon
Professor of Early Childhood Intervention, Department Family, Child and Social Work, MSH Medical School, Hamburg, Germany

Stefanus Snyman
Research associate, Centre for Community Technologies, Nelson Mandela University, Port Elizabeth, South Africa; Project Manager, WHO-FIC Collaborating Centre for the Africa Region, South African Medical Research Council, Cape Town, South Africa.

Hillegonda A Stallinga
Researcher, University of Groningen, University Medical Center Groningen, Department of Health Sciences, Section Nursing Research, Groningen, the Netherlands

Introduction

Peter L Rosenbaum

From time to time in the field of healthcare an exciting new development appears on the horizon to challenge and potentially transform thinking and behaviour. Changes may involve new approaches to the provision of care; the education of health professionals; how research is conceptualised and conducted; the organisation of services; and sometimes additional ideas not originally envisioned by the people who started the process. Often, in fact, changes in one area beget unexpected changes elsewhere. The contributors to this handbook on the World Health Organization's (WHO's) International Classification of Functioning, Disability and Health (ICF) (Fifty-Fourth World Health Assembly 2001, World Health Organization 2001) and its Children and Youth Version (ICF-CY; World Health Organization 2007) believe that the ICF represents one of those transformative resources that bear closer examination.

The predecessor of this book was published in German (Kraus de Camargo & Simon 2013) by two of the editors of this book as a collection of thoughts and experiences derived from many workshops provided since 2007, with the launch of the ICF-CY, to a variety of professionals in the field of Early Childhood Intervention and Developmental Paediatrics. In the process of translating it into English, we recognized that many changes had occurred in the intervening years that warranted a deeper and more detailed description of the underpinnings of 'ICF thinking'. We were also very aware of developments around the world in clinical practice. We have been particularly interested in the restructuring of the curriculums for healthcare professionals to include the philosophy, the framework and the tools offered by the ICF. Many of the practical examples from the original book have been kept as the questions addressed and the way of approaching solutions seem to us universal and applicable to any location.

Background

The ICF is a World Health Organization initiative (2001) that is increasingly widely used – especially in the field of childhood disability. The framework for health is, in the view of the authors, an excellent model for all health professionals and should, we believe, be introduced to all health profession students from the outset of their education. There are several features of the ICF, listed in the following sections, that we hope to highlight in this handbook that readers will find both useful and applicable.

Using the ICF as a conceptual framework

The ICF attributes offer a conceptual framework for health; these are outlined in Chapters 1–4. Key ideas that we find compelling include that the ICF provides:

- a biopsychosocial framework – illustrating the integration and interaction of the biological and social models of health into a unitary framework;

- a holistic approach to health – applies to the whole person, and to every person;

- a strength-based model – emphasising functioning;

- a theoretical premise of universalism (disability as a human trait), thus enforcing Human Rights for everybody including People with Disabilities (UN 2006);

- neutral language, modelling an approach towards people's strengths;

- aetiologic neutrality and parity – which applies to all health issues;

- an interactional (dynamic) structure (with 'disability' as a potential outcome when there is a misfit among elements of people's lives);

- multidimensionality and comprehensiveness.

As the ICF is grounded in UN Conventions of the Rights of Children and of People with Disabilities, it provides a framework for considering the ethical dimensions of all health encounters and practices. For example, is impairment alone responsible for disability (stigma, social isolation, poor education or poor housing)?

The ICF is a versatile tool

The ICF is a tool with multiple potential applications (Chapters 5–8)

These potential applications include:

- A personalised clinical documentation and organisational tool for patients (and practitioners) to identify strengths, problems/issues, needs and goals, and to help identify windows for management and evaluations of specific management.

- A tool to explore and explicate issues of people's vulnerability.

- Educational tools for all health professions, with respect to thinking about health in a broader context than the biomedical dimensions of health and disease alone.

- A terminology and communication tool: Classificatory, international and interprofessional.

- An epidemiological tool to collect and analyse data.

- An ethical tool (promoting the central values of respect, confidentiality, autonomy, beneficence, benevolence and justice/fairness).

- A health policy tool.

This book has been created by clinician educators and health services researchers who work primarily in the field of Child and Youth Developmental healthcare (disability). Its purpose is to share with readers the ways in which we perceive that the ICF has fundamentally changed and enhanced our field, and how it has the potential to have similar impacts well beyond this particular area of healthcare. We see opportunities for the ICF framework and concepts to improve interprofessional communication and collaboration across all areas of health services, most particularly, but not limited to, chronic care. Throughout the book, we draw on and report both the literature and our experiences in practice, teaching, research and writing to illustrate the potential ways in which ICF ideas may be useful to others – whoever they are in the complex world of healthcare. The book is not meant to be either prescriptive or a 'how-to' manual; rather we aim to offer insights into the ways that all of our activities in healthcare can be reconsidered through this new and dynamic lens.

The book consists of three sections. The four chapters in Section A discuss conceptual issues that provide a context and background to the ICF. Chapter 1 introduces the ICF and offers a perspective on the evolving concept of health in the current century. It describes how we are moving from thinking about a health condition as a biomedical problem that resides within the anatomy or physiology of the person (often established clinically by 'ruling out' competing diagnostic considerations) to a biopsychosocial framework that formally encompassed personal and environmental factors, and actively 'rules in' elements of a person's life that may impact their health and hence provide 'points of entry' for interventions. Chapter 2 discusses the idea of 'functioning' as the central notion in modern ideas about conceptualising 'health'. In Chapter 3, two ICF concepts are discussed in detail. 'Personal factors' are one of the 'contextual' elements of the ICF that are now explicitly meant to be identified and used in the formulation of a person's story. The second component of Chapter 3 is a discussion of the idea of 'participation' – engagement in life in ways that are meaningful and important to a person. In many ways participation is the pinnacle of health, insofar as one is able to realise one's personal 'engagement' regardless of how those activities are accomplished. The last chapter of this section of the book (Chapter 4) explores the relationship between patient/person-reported outcomes (PROs) and the ICF. Ideas in this chapter illustrate how, at both the clinical and the research level, this essentially personal valuation of one's life is very important to understand, and complementary to professionals' evaluations of our interventions based solely on clinicians' and researchers' ideas about how a disease or disorder, and the impact of interventions, should be measured.

The four chapters in Section B present readers with examples of ways to operationalise the ICF language and concepts in several areas of clinical life. In Chapter 5 the authors illustrate how the ICF can be used in everyday clinical practice and offer the reader the opportunity to try out these ideas with case examples. Moving beyond the immediate clinical 'case', Chapter 6 describes the value of an ICF-informed team for promoting effective health and social care. Chapter 7 describes ways that the ICF framework, language and concepts should inform the fundamental education and acculturation of all health professionals – a goal we believe can and must be achieved. The last chapter in this section (Chapter 8) discusses the value of using the ICF concepts to inform the policies, administration and advocacy efforts of clinical and health services programs.

Section C offers two chapters with specific perspectives on the ICF. In Chapter 9 the voice of an informed parent of a child with complex special needs is heard as she reflects on how the ICF concepts and language might have been very useful to her and her family had these ideas been available in the 1990s when she was on her own very challenging journey with her son. Chapter 10 provides a speculative view, looking forward and considering potential future developments and uses of the ICF.

The 10 chapters of this book provide overviews of concepts that are designed to introduce the ICF and to report the many ways that people are applying the ICF ideas in their work – be it for clinical, research or administrative purposes. At the end of the book we have also included seven appendices that offer a deeper dive into the issues discussed in the text. These materials, which include case examples and exercises, team development phases etc. provide readers with opportunities to 'try out' and to apply the ideas that this book promotes. These are simply a few specific illustrations of the ways people may want to use the ICF concepts and the tools that are being developed to implement these ideas in their own orbit. Appendix 3 illustrates one of the tools that have been created to bring the 'F-words in childhood disability' to life. The F-words, discussed elsewhere in the book, provide a tongue-in-cheek approach as to how to operationalize the ICF concepts; the links in Appendix 7 direct the reader to the F-words hub on the CanChild website, where they will find a host of clinical tools that allow people to use these ideas in ways that have been shown to appeal to – in fact to have been developed with and by – parents and young people with impairments as well as to service providers and program managers. Readers may choose to use these materials for group exercises within their clinical or research teams to promote a common understanding of the application of the ICF to their specific needs.

Caveats

It is of course important to note what the ICF does not do! First, while the framework provides a structure into which to aggregate the details of an individual's current health reality across several dimensions, the resulting profile provides only a point-in-time snapshot account of that person's situation. There is no temporal element to the profile, meaning that as the person's story evolves it is essential to update the profile.

Second, the profile provides a factual account of the person's situation, objectively described, measured or perceived, with little or no valuation of the details. Even the contextual elements of personal and environmental factors are meant to provide perspectives on these aspects of people's lives but not how people value these components. That is done – or in our view should be done – using the fully-populated ICF framework as the 'raw material' with which to identify both the issues of importance to a person or their family, and the potential strategies to approach those issues.

A corollary to this idea is that the ICF framework does not provide an account of people's 'quality of life' – at least not what we refer to as the existential perspectives of people's personal valuation of their life quality. There are other more focused approaches to 'quality of life' – 'health-related', social determinants and econometric systems – that could potentially use the details in a populated ICF framework to calculate, for example, a health 'utility' value based on an individual's functional profile (Torrance 1987). Once again, however, such a value would not include how people feel about or self-evaluate their lives. This is important because it has been shown that even when people have what might objectively be assumed to be 'severe disability' they may still adapt to a new health situation and self-assess their quality of life to be very good (Albrecht & Devlieger 1999).

Users of the ICF need to be aware of these limitations and always document ICF information collaboratively with the patient and their family (and other professionals involved in the care) to obtain the best possible understanding of what matters to the patient and their family.

This book is meant to introduce the ICF as a tool to expand our thinking and actions across all dimensions of the field of healthcare. The authors have taken every opportunity to illuminate the concepts we present with examples from our own work and that of others to illustrate the rich opportunities to rethink and improve healthcare, made possible by this biopsychosocial framework. Needless to say, feedback from colleagues who read and use this book will enrich our understanding of the ICF and of those areas of our presentation of the ICF ideas that are not as clear as we hoped!

References

Albrecht GL, Devlieger PJ (1999) The disability paradox: High quality of life against all odds. *Soc Sci Med* **48**: 977–988.

Fifty-Fourth World Health Assembly (2001) *International Classification of Functioning Disability and Health (ICF). Resolution WHA54.21*. Geneva, 14–22 May.

Kraus de Camargo O, Simon L (2013) *Die ICF-CY in der Praxis [Practical use of the ICF-CY]*. Bern: Verlag Hans Huber.

Torrance GW (1987) Utility approach to measuring health-related quality of life. *J Chron Dis* **40**(6): 593–603.

WHO (World Health Organization) (1980) *International Classification of Impairments Disabilities and Handicaps*. Geneva: World Health Organization.

WHO (World Health Organization) (1992) *International Statistical Classification of Diseases and Related Health Problems 10th Revision (ICD-10), 10th edn*. Geneva: World Health Organization.

WHO (World Health Organization) (2001) *International Classification of Functioning Disability and Health: ICF*. Geneva: World Health Organization.

WHO (World Health Organization) (2007) *International Classification of Functioning Disability and Health – Children and Youth Version, 1st edn*. Geneva: World Health Organization.

Section A

Chapter 1

The ICF and the biopsychosocial model of health: From 'disease' to 'health condition'

Olaf Kraus de Camargo

The foundations of modern biomedicine are based on the recognition that biological processes underlie clinical findings and symptoms presented by the patient. One of the founders of this scientific biomedical approach is Rudolf Karl Virchow (1821–1902) with his seminal work on cellular pathology published in 1847 (Benaroyo 1998).

Interestingly, Virchow is also considered to be the founder of 'social medicine', having coined the phrase 'medicine is a social science'. He recognised, with the same scientific acumen that guided his pathology studies, that the fight against epidemics that were rampant at his time in Europe (e.g. typhus) could only be successful with social change improving living conditions, especially of the poorer population (Virchow 1848). At almost the same time (1854) Dr John Snow (1813–1858) was tracing the source of the cholera epidemic in London to the water supply by drawing a systematic map of Soho where the victims of cholera died. His work led to separate water systems for clean and waste. The story is compellingly told by Steven Johnson (2006).

The 19th century was the period when people first began to collect information on diseases in a systematic way, notably with the work of the medical statisticians William Farr (1807–1883) in the UK and Jacques Bertillon (1851–1922) in France. In August 1900, the French government organised the first conference to review the 'International Classification of Causes of Death'. This was followed by a succession of conferences during the 20th century, particularly with the aim of fighting the epidemics of cholera, typhoid and smallpox. In 1923, an International Health Organization was established in Geneva but only in 1948 did it become the international body that today is known as the World Health Organization (WHO; World Health Organization 2012). Although it had its origins in meetings and conferences with a focus on death rates and their statistics, the WHO eventually developed into a worldwide organisation with the broad aim of improving the general health of populations.

This change of perspective is also reflected in the expansion of the classification systems developed by the WHO, and it characterises a shift in the conceptual understanding of the relationship between disease and health. Initially, taxonomies such as the International Classification of Diseases (ICD) were based on a biomedical model of disease; this later expanded to include information about psychological and social determinants of health, and reflected the adoption of the biopsychosocial model of health, which was recognised to be better fitted to the need to represent and describe the many aspects of people's lives as part of a broader definition of health (Engel 1977).

In the **biomedical model**, ill health is seen as a problem that arises directly from diseases, trauma or other health problems, and is situated within the person. The care required to treat an ill person is provided by health professionals, whose goal is to achieve healing with treatments or surgeries, adaptation to the condition if it is not curable, and behavioural changes of the individual.

The WHO's **biopsychosocial framework for health** – the International Classification of Functioning, Disability and Health (ICF) (2001) – grew out of the WHO's (1980) development of the International Classification of Impairments, Disabilities and Handicaps (ICIDH). With the input of colleagues around the world, and the perspectives of people with disabilities, the ICIDH was revised and updated by the WHO to better describe the effects and the interactions of the context with a person's life on their health. This classification was endorsed in 2001 by the 191 Member States of the WHO (Fifty-Fourth World Health Assembly 2001). Since 2007, the Children and Youth Version (ICF-CY) has been available in English (WHO 2007). In this book, the abbreviation 'ICF' relates to general statements about the framework and classification, and the abbreviation 'CY' refers specifically to the version for children and young people. Figure 1.1 shows the ICF framework, illustrating the several elements of the ICF and the interconnectedness of the parts to one another.

In the **biopsychosocial model**, representing 21st century thinking, health is conceptualised as a person's functioning within a context. A problem of functional health (see Chapter 3) can be caused by both intrinsic biomedical disorders, and external contextual factors impacting on the person. Consequently, helping to improve functional health is not a domain restricted to healthcare professionals. The goals for functional health can include the options described above, but also involve identification and

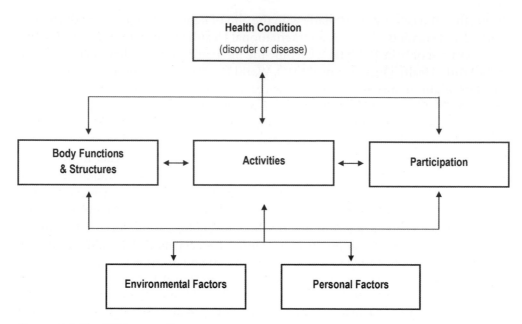

Figure 1.1 The ICF framework
Reprinted from WHO 2001, p. 18, © 2001.

removal of legal, physical and societal/social barriers to achieving full integration of the affected person into society. Examples of barriers include the obvious physical challenges of access for people with functional challenges of, for example, vision or mobility, as well as less apparent attitudinal factors that limit employment and social opportunities for people with impairments. By contrast, facilitators can include a host of workplace and school accommodations beyond the 'usual' physical access to enable people who need these to work and study during flexible hours, or from home, and facilitate their access to transportation. Further facilitators are technical aids, such as voice recognition software, that help people communicate effectively based on intellectual ability rather than on physical limitations, In this way of understanding, 'restricted functional health' is not a characteristic of a person, but is seen as a complex set of interconnected conditions, many of which are created by the social environment and frequently require social action. It is the collective responsibility of society to shape the environment in a way that allows the full participation of people with health problems in all areas of social life.

With reference to human wellbeing, anthropology plays a fundamental role in theories regarding therapeutic interventions. In addition to the cognitive, the conative, the affective and bodily dimension of our being human, spirituality should be viewed as a coherence factor that deals with purposefulness and meaning. It contributes to wholeness as an expression of hope and an intimate sense of belongingness (Louw 2016).

Huber et al. (2016) demonstrated that patients value the aspect of spirituality as an important component of health. The person-centred use of the ICF leads to an expanded view of the biopsychosocial model, called a bio-psycho-social-spiritual approach (De Villiers et al. 2014, World Health Organization 2013).

To do justice to these psychological and environmental factors, the ICF – as well as the ICF-CY – is divided into two major parts: (1): Functioning and Disability, and (2): Contextual Factors. Functioning and Disability is further divided into: a) Body Functions and Structures, and b) Activities and Participation. Contextual Factors are also further divided into: a) Environmental Factors and b) Personal Factors. Each of these four components in turn is subdivided into individual chapters, in which the user finds sub-categories (items) that aim to describe, as fully as possible, all variations and aspects of functional health (see the Functional health section). For example, the chapter on Communication is a component of Activities and Participation and has, among others, the items d330 Speaking and d345 Writing Messages.

The practical application of the ICF is based on the identification of those items that most comprehensively and accurately describe the individual situation of a person at the current time, in order to be able to provide the best possible support and treatment relevant to current strengths, issues, realities and challenges. This manual is designed to help with this task.

Functional health

This central concept of the ICF is defined as follows:

A person is considered *functionally healthy* if, taking in account their entire life background (concept of Contextual Factors):

- their bodily functions (including cognitive functions) and body structures correspond to generally accepted standards (concepts of Body Functions and Structures),

- they do or can do activities of the type and to the full extent as is expected from a person without any health problem (concept of Activities), and

- they can develop their existence in all areas of life that are important to them, in the way that a person without impairments of body functions/structures and activity limitations would do (concept of Participation).

In consequence, and as a corollary, *disability* is defined as a negative interaction between a person (whose health condition may correspond to the definition of an ICD-coded diagnosis) and the contextual factors that affect the person's functioning (Leonardi et al. 2006).

Specifically, a disability is present when this negative interaction impacts the person's participation in specific life areas (e.g. in the nursery, school, play, work or leisure activities) that are important to them. Disabilities are thus not absolute, nor do they reside within the person, but are relative to life areas and the 'fit' between person and environment (Leonardi et al. 2006).

The division of the Contextual Factors into Environmental Factors and Personal Factors serves to remind us that the activities that are important for an individual also depend on personal inclinations and interests, rather than being about the fulfilment of absolute standards. Personal Factors are not classified into items and coded, because they may strongly depend on cultural as well as personal values (see Chapter 3).

To allow a better description of functional health in infants and young children, the Child and Youth version of the ICF-CY contains numerous additional child and youth-specific categories in the areas of Body Functions and Structures, Activities and Participation as well as in the Contextual Factors, many of which have been integrated into ICF 2017. This work of updating the ICF is an ongoing task supported by the Functioning and Disability Reference Group (FDRG) of the World Health Organization Family of International Classifications (WHO-FIC Network http://www.who.int/classifications/network/).

In relation to the components of health, some definitions have been established by the WHO:

- Body functions are the physiological functions of body systems (including psychological functions).
- Body structures are anatomical parts of the body such as organs, limbs and their components.
- Impairments are problems in body function or structure such as a significant deviation or loss.
- Activity is the execution of a task or action by an individual.
- Participation is involvement in a life situation.
- Activity limitations are difficulties an individual may have in executing activities.
- Participation restrictions are problems an individual may experience in involvement in life situations.
- Environmental factors make up the physical, social and attitudinal environment in which people live and conduct their lives.
- Personal factors are a particular background of an individual's life and living, and comprise features of the individual that are not part of a health condition or health states (WHO 2007).

The goals of intervention planning should be based on the possibilities for children to engage in activity and participation in their environment. The German Association for Early Intervention explicitly calls for a systematic use of the ICF-CY in order to capture relevant information and obtain a view of the health status of children within their contexts (ViFF (Vereinigung für Interdisziplinare Frühförderung) 2003; 2009). Such a detailed presentation can be useful for family- and patient-centred planning of support, therapies and assistance. Making use of the ICF allows people to capture the needs expressed by patients and families and also those identified by different professionals. This information, using a common framework and language, facilitates the process of shared decision-making when determining the most urgent needs to be addressed.

The consequence of using the ICF for intervention planning (therapy, early intervention, counselling and coaching) is that the goals are not necessarily related to the 'normalisation' of specific body functions. The goals of individual families and children might be very distinct and will need to be addressed within their specific contexts. These individualised intervention goals might be operationalised using tools such as the Canadian Occupational Performance Measure (COPM) (Law et al. 2005, McColl et al. 2005), and the Perceived Efficacy and Goal Setting (PEGS) tool (Missiuna et al. 2006). Tools like these are designed to take into account daily activities of children and their expectations, and allow people setting these goals to define meaningful targets from the perspective of the person with the health need rather than the professional.

The Participation and Environment Measure for Children and Youth (PEM-CY) is a recent measure developed to assess participation and contextual factors when planning for the rehabilitation of children and young people. It is a good example of the modern tools that are being developed based on the principles of the ICF (Coster et al. 2012) (see https://www.canchild.ca/en/resources/248-participation-and-environment-measure-for-children-and-youth-pem-cy).

Core sets and checklists

In contrast to the ICD, which has specific codes for specific diagnoses like epilepsy, cerebral palsy, obesity, traumatic brain injury or emotional disorders, the ICF codes are not specific for distinct diagnoses or conditions. This reflects the non-categorical nature of the ICF (meaning that none of the ICF ideas is diagnosis-specific). It is possible, however, to select a number of codes that might require more attention when dealing with a certain diagnosis. This approach is similar to the process when taking a clinical history: after initial general questions, we start to ask more specific questions according to the condition suspected, in order to confirm it ('rule it in') or move it lower in probability ('rule it out'). If the ICF codes that are common to a certain diagnosis are collected in a systematic way, the result can be aggregated into a 'set' or a group of codes coming from various domains of the ICF, such as Body Functions, Body

Structures, Activities and Participation and Environmental Factors. Such groupings are called 'Core sets',as they are believed to represent core elements common to most patients with a defined diagnosis. Many core sets have been developed over the years for adults, following a standardised procedure (Selb et al. 2015). They exist for patients with multiple sclerosis, bipolar disorders and cancer, to name a few (Bickenbach et al. 2012). In the paediatric field, there is still very little experience using core sets. They have been developed for cerebral palsy and for autism spectrum disorders (Schiariti & Masse 2014, Bölte et al. 2014). Over 10 years ago, at the University Hospital in Freiburg, Germany, the Department for Child and Youth Psychiatry used a subset of items for planning purposes and environmental assessment of patients with diagnoses such as autism, attention-deficit–hyperactivity disorder and eating disorders (Kolch et al. 2007). In the field of Early Intervention, using a checklist with age-specific categories (not diagnosis-specific) was proposed in Germany (Kraus de Camargo 2007, Kaffka-Backmann et al. 2007).

The use of core sets, questionnaires and tests is common practice in medicine. Nonetheless, a narrative approach can add details and richness not captured with standardised tools. Relying exclusively on a core set to determine a person's functional level can lead people to miss important individual needs (Grötzbach & Iven 2009, p. 25). It also seems to the contributors to this book that the idea of 'core sets' can easily appear to run counter to the basic notion of the openness to an individualised approach with an ICF 'profile' as an intrinsically important function of thinking in this ICF-based way.

To understand functional health, especially of younger children, it is important to be aware that relying only on the description of problems and identifying which of the components of the ICF they correspond to might not help in planning for the best support. The context, the family and personal factors, and an understanding of their interactions with other components form such an integrated and interwoven unit in early childhood that the isolation of single factors often does not make much sense (Hollenweger 2009, p. 205).

All attempts to use 'Core sets' or 'Checklists' to facilitate the use of the ICF-CY need to be undertaken with the recognition that the purpose of using the ICF is to describe the functioning of a person with all their unique and individual aspects (in other words, 'rule in' relevant features), rather than to make a diagnosis. It is therefore important to have categories available that, though they might not be typical or frequent in the population of a certain health condition, are relevant for the individual that is being assessed and described. This is particularly the case with environmental factors, both, barriers and facilitators, might vary hugely from one region, and one person, to another. In the future, we expect that functional profiles using the ICF will be created with information technology that allows a greater direct and empowering involvement of people themselves in that process (Snyman et al. 2015).

To avoid the diagnostic specificity of 'core sets' and the associated labelling of such an approach, the German Working Group for the Implementation of the ICF-CY developed age-related Checklists for the ICF-CY that are shorter than the full ICF-CY and can make it easier to use the ICF in those populations. Those age-related lists are available in German on the websites of the participating member associations of the working group, and an English version is found in Appendix 6 of this book, available to download from the Mac Keith Press website or in e-versions (Deutsche Interdisziplinäre Arbeitsgruppe zur ICF Adaptation für den Kinder – und Jugendbereich 2012).

Evaluation of interventions

When children with chronic health conditions or developmental disabilities receive interventions that were planned according to the concept of the ICF-CY, it becomes necessary and important to document the effects and results of such interventions using the ICF. One approach is to use Goal Attainment Scaling (GAS).

GAS is not a specific standardised tool but an approach that is easy to implement in rehabilitation as well as in other settings (McDougall & Wright 2009, Steenbeek et al. 2007). GAS starts with defining a goal with the child/parents, as well as the time frame after which this goal should be reached. At the relevant time after intervention, one determines the degree to which the goal has been attained. A critical aspect of such an approach is often that the process of defining goals might be challenging for children. It might also be challenging to negotiate the potential discrepancies of goals between child and parents or between partners. On the other hand, it is worthwhile and important to be aware of such discrepant expectations and to address them at the beginning of the intervention process. In fact, it is desirable to identify such discrepancies at the beginning of an intervention rather than to try to understand, a posteriori, what the reason might be for apparent 'failure' or 'non-compliance' after the intervention did not attain the established goals.

The PEGS (see Core sets and Checklists section) can be used not only for intervention planning, but also for evaluating such interventions. Another tool is the CAPE (Children's Assessment of Participation and Enjoyment) (King et al. 2007), which is validated for children and young people from the ages 6–21 years. It consists of 55 questions related to their activities of daily living and their preferences. This tool is not designed to measure the quality of performance in executing a certain activity. Rather, the goal is to determine if children are enabled to participate in activities that they prefer, or increase the number of activities in which they are able to participate.

The different ways of describing participation are gaining more importance in the evaluation of early intervention and rehabilitation. The ICF can help to operationalise such an approach by identifying the relevant areas to be assessed, but also to select the appropriate instruments for the assessment. To be able to do this, instruments need to be mapped to the ICF, so they can reveal which components of the ICF are being assessed. For example, the 'Kidscreen/Disabkids' is a collection of questionnaires to assess biopsychosocial health and quality of life, developed by partners in the European Union and available in many languages (Dutch, English, French, German, Greek, Norwegian, Swedish) (https://www.kidscreen.org/english/project/; https://www.disabkids.org). A content analysis of the measure revealed that many questions relate to the Activities and Participation components of the ICF (Fayed et al. 2012).

By no means will 'classic' evaluation tools that measure changes at the level of body structures and functions become obsolete, but in order to be appreciated those detailed accounts of specific functions need to be seen within the larger concept and context of functional health. A detailed overview of clinical measures for the assessment and evaluation of the care of children with developmental disabilities, and their relation to the ICF, can be found in the book *Measures for Children with Developmental Disability: an ICF-CY approach* (Majnemer 2012).

References

Benaroyo L (1998) Rudolf Virchow and the scientific approach to medicine. *Endeavour* **22**(3): 114–116.

Bickenbach J,Cieza A,Rauch A,Stucki G (2012) ICF-based documentation tool – ICF core sets in clinical practice [online]. http://www.icf-core-sets.org.

Bölte S, De Schipper E, Robison JE, et al. (2014) Classification of functioning and impairment: The development of ICF core sets for autism spectrum disorder. *Autism Res* **7**(1): 167–172.

Coster W, Law M, Bedell G, Khetani M, Cousins M, Teplicky R (2012) Development of the participation and environment measure for children and youth: conceptual basis. *Disabil Rehabil* **34**(3): 238–246.

De Villiers M, Conradie H, Snyman S, Van Heerden B, Van Schalkwyk S (2014) Experiences in developing and implementing a community-based education strategy – A case study from South Africa. In: Talaat W, Ladhani L (eds.) *Community-Based Education in Health Professions: Global Perspectives*. Cairo: World Health Organization Regional Office for the Eastern Mediterranean, pp. 176–206.

Deutsche Interdisziplinare Arbeitsgruppe zur ICF Adaptation für den Kinder – und Jugendbereich (2012) ICF-CY Checklists [online]. http://www.bvkm.de/servicematerialien/icf-checklisten-kinder-und-jugendliche-fuer-die-praxis-aufbereitet.html.

Engel GL (1977) The need for a new medical model: a challenge for biomedicine. *Science* **196**(4286): 129–136.

Fayed N, Kraus de Camargo O, Kerr E, et al. (2012) Generic patient-reported outcomes in child health research: A review of conceptual content using World Health Organization definitions. *Dev Med Child Neurol* **54**(12):1085–1095.

Fifty-Fourth World Health Assembly (2001) *International Classification of Functioning Disability and Health (ICF). Resolution WHA54.21*. Geneva, 14–22 May.

Grötzbach H, Iven C (eds.) (2009) *ICF in der Sprachförderung*. Idstein: Schulz-Kirchner Verlag.

Hollenweger J (2009) ICF in der Frühförderung. In: Grötzbach H, Iven C (eds.) *ICF in der Sprach-förderung.* Idstein: Schulz-Kirchner Verlag.

Huber M van Vliet M, Giezenberg M, et al. (2016) Towards a 'patient-centred' operationalisation of the new dynamic concept of health: a mixed methods study. *BMJ Open* **6**(1): e010091.

Johnson S (2006) *The Ghost Map: The Story of London's Most Terrifying Epidemic – And How it Changed Science Cities and the Modern World.* Penguin Random House.

Kaffka-Backmann M, Simon L, Grunwaldt A (2007) Praktische Erfahrungen mit der Verwendung einer ICF-Checkliste für die Interdisziplinare Frühförderung ('ICF-Checkliste IFF'). *Frühförderung Interdisziplinär* **26**(4): 167–172.

King GA, Law M, King S, et al. (2007) Measuring children's participation in recreation and leisure activities: construct validation of the CAPE and PAC. *Child Care Health Dev* **33**(1): 28–39.

Kolch M, Wolff M, Fegert JM (2007) Teilhabebeeinträchtigung-Möglichkeiten der Standardisierung im Verfahren nach § 35a SGB VII. *Das Jugendamt* **1**: 1–8.

Kraus de Camargo O (2007) Die ICF-CY als Checkliste und Dokumentationsraster in der Praxis der Frühförderung. *Frühförderung Interdisziplinär* **26**: 158–166.

Law M, Baptiste S, Carswell A, McColl MA, Polatajko HJ, Pollock N (2005) The Canadian Occupational Performance Measure: an outcome measure for occupational therapy. *Can J Occup Ther* **57**(2): 82–87.

Leonardi M, Bickenbach J, Ustun TB, Kostanjsek N, Chatterji S, Consortium M (2006) The definition of disability: what is in a name? Lancet **368**: 1219–1221.

Louw DJ (2016) Wholeness in spiritual healing and helping. towards a base anthropology for a pastoral hermeneutics of hope care. In: *Wholeness in Hope Care. On Nurturing the Beauty of the Human Soul in Spiritual Healing.* Berlin: Lit Verlag, pp. 1–22.

Majnemer A (ed.) (2012) *Measures for Children with Developmental Disability: An ICF-CY Approach.* London: Mac Keith Press.

McColl MA, Law M, Baptiste S, et al. (2005) Targeted applications of the Canadian Occupational Performance Measure. *Can J Occ Ther* **72**(5): 298–300.

McDougall J, Wright V (2009) The ICF-CY and Goal Attainment Scaling: benefits of their combined use for pediatric practice. *Disabil Rehabil* **31**(16): 1362–1372.

Missiuna C, Pollock N, Law M, Walter S, Cavey N (2006) Examination of the perceived efficacy and goal setting system (PEGS) with children with disabilities their parents and teachers. *Am J Occ Ther* **60**: 204–214.

Schiariti V, Masse LC (2014) Relevant areas of functioning in children with cerebral palsy based on the International Classification of Functioning Disability and Health Coding System: A clinical perspective. *J Child Neurol* **30**(2): 216–222.

Selb M, Escorpizo R, Kostanjsek N, Stucki G, Ustun TB, Cieza A (2015) A guide on how to develop an International Classification of Functioning Disability and Health Core Set. *Eur J Phys Rehabil Med* **51**(1): 105–117.

Snyman S, Kraus de Camargo O, Welch Saleeby P, Paltamaa J, Anttila H (2015) Mobile application for the ICF International Classification of Functioning Disability and Health (mICF). *13th Congress of European Forum for Research in Rehabilitation.* Helsinki, Finland, p. 49.

Steenbeek D, Ketelaar M, Galama K, Gorter JW (2007) Goal attainment scaling in paediatric rehabilitation: a critical review of the literature. *Dev Med Child Neurol* **49**: 550–556.

ViFF (Vereinigung für Interdisziplinare Frühförderung) (2003) *Handreichungen zur inter-disziplinären Diagnostik zur Erstellung eines Förder – und Behandlungsplanes und des Zugangs zur Komplexleistung Früherkennung und Frühförderung.* Munich: Vereinigung für Interdisziplinare Frühförderung.

ViFF (Vereinigung für Interdisziplinäre Frühförderung) (2009) *Empfehlungen zur Diagnostik im Rahmen der Komplexleistung in Interdisziplinären Frühförderstellen.* Munich: Vereinigung für Inter-disziplinare Frühförderung.

Virchow RC (1848) *Mittheilungen über die in Oberschlesien herrschende Typhus-Epidemie.* Archiv für path Anat u Physiol u für klin Medicin. Berlin: G. Reimer.

WHO (World Health Organization) (2001) *International Classification of Functioning Disability and Health: ICF.* Geneva: World Health Organization.

WHO (World Health Organization) (2007) *International Classification of Functioning Disability and Health – Children and Youth Version, 1st edn.* Geneva: World Health Organization.

WHO (World Health Organization) (2012) History of the WHO [online]. *WHO Historical Collection.* http://www.who.int/about/history/en/.

WHO (World Health Organization) (2013) *How to Use the ICF: A Practical Manual for Using the International Classification of Functioning Disability and Health (ICF).* Geneva: World Health Organization.

Chapter 2
The concept of 'functioning'
Hillegonda A Stallinga

Introduction

Why is it relevant to write about the concept of 'functioning' in the context of the ICF? First, functioning is the central theme of the ICF – the International Classification of Functioning, Disability and Health, published by the World Health Organization (WHO) in 2001. Second, the idea of functioning can easily be ambiguous. Since the ICF first appeared, it has been people's experience that using the ICF, including the unified linguistic terms for aspects of functioning, does not necessarily mean that the concept of functioning is understood the same way by those using it (Chou & Kröger 2017). This chapter provides an overview of descriptions and models related to the concept of functioning; discusses when people are functioning successfully; and points out why and how to use the concept of functioning as a major focus for healthcare.

What is meant by the concept of functioning

Descriptions of the concept of functioning

The WHO describes 'functioning' in the ICF as an umbrella term encompassing all body functions, structures, activities and participation; similarly, 'disability' serves as an umbrella term for impairments, activity limitations and participation restrictions (WHO 2001). Functioning must be understood as a result of a dynamic interaction between the health condition and contextual factors (e.g. environmental and personal factors). Furthermore, functioning has to be seen as a continuous concept, that is, a concept that is 'more or less', and measurable along a continuum rang-ing from completely able to completely disabled (Bickenbach et al. 2012, Stallinga 2015). Finally, the ICF distinguishes two constructs: 'capacity' and 'performance', specifically applicable for the components of activities and participation to express one's functioning. Capacity is defined as 'an individual's ability to execute a task or an action'; performance is defined as 'what an individual does in his or her current environment' (WHO 2001).

In recent published documents, the WHO also uses the term 'functional ability'. Functional ability refers to:

> the attributes that enable people to be and to do what they have reason to value. It is determined by individuals' intrinsic capacity (the combination of all their physical and mental – including psychosocial – capacities), the environments they inhabit and the interaction between the individual and these environments (WHO 2017).

Functional ability seems to be closely related to functioning as described above in the context of the ICF. All the components of the ICF are included. However, the difference with the ICF is the broadened description of the term 'capacity' by including 'what they have valued'. That, in turn, is closely related to the term 'capability' as described in the Capability Approach of Amartya Sen (Sen 1992). In Sen's interpretation, capability is defined as 'the availability of realistic opportunities to do or become what one has chosen' and is somewhat similar to the term functioning (Sen 1992). Functioning is defined as 'the "beings and doings" a person achieves, chosen by an individual by using his/her capabilities' (Sen 1992). A difference between the ICF and Capability Approach is that the latter is a political–theoretical account of egalitarian justice, whereas the ICF is meant only as a classification system for describing functioning in the context of health (Bickenbach 2014). Bickenbach demonstrated that a comparison of the Capability Approach and the ICF reveals salient aspects of convergence that arguably point to a potential synergy between both approaches when it comes to the conceptualisation of functioning (Bickenbach 2014). From the Capability Approach, we can appreciate that lacking the 'capability to convert resources into genuine and realistic opportunities to pursue goals and life plans' will decrease one's level of functioning as described in the ICF (Bickenbach 2014).

Similarities among all the listed descriptions of functioning can be found in the con-ceptualisation of functioning as a whole. No single aspect determines functioning. The concept of functioning has to be considered as an entity, capturing all that people *have* (body functions and body structures, e.g. sensory functions, eyes), all that people *do* (activities, e.g. tasks, skills) and all that people *are or aspire to be* (participation, e.g. being a parent, being an employee) (Bickenbach et al. 2012).

The concept of functioning and the Biopsychosocial Model

In order to capture the integration of the various aspects of functioning, the 'biopsychosocial' model is used in the ICF's theoretical base. The initial biopsychosocial model was introduced by Engel (1977). This model is considered as a complex, adaptive, personal, and experiential systems model. The main characteristic, as in many other systems models (General Systems Theory) is that no single characteristic alone is responsible for the level of an individual's functioning. This means that the system can fail even if all subparts are intact and working properly (Wade & Halligan 2017). Think of a flock of birds: every bird can fly separately, but to be a flock means that each bird has to interact in the right position at the right time. Applied to the ICF, even the presence of all functions, structures, activities and participation items represented in the ICF categories does not necessarily lead to people having successful functioning. On the other hand, deviation of one aspect, e.g. having a severe limitation in walking, does not necessarily mean that someone cannot function successfully. The biopsychosocial model attempts to achieve a synthesis, in order to provide a coherent view of different perspectives related to health from a biological, individual (personal) and social perspective (Wade & Halligan 2017). The person can determine for him or herself whether the various components are in balance (Sturmberg 2009, Wade & Halligan 2017). That implies that the health or social care professional, as a user of the ICF, must always take into consideration all the components of the model in relation to each other and the relationships among them – always in collaboration with the individual's goals and values – to try to improve functioning. It is the whole person, viewed in a holistic way, with their resources, (dis)abilities in their physical, attitudinal, social, and political environment, that has to be taken into account.

When are people functioning successfully?

The ICF provides opportunities to describe people's status of functioning both from the perspective of professionals (what is assumed to be an 'objective' view) and from the perspective of the person themselves (what is assumed to be the perceived subjective assessment). Functioning is critically centred on the individual's complex systems, including medical factors and personal factors, in interaction (really in transaction) with their physical environment in a goal-directed way and over time. In that way, successful functioning can be described as achieving one's personal goals by properly managing one's physical, psychological, sociological and contextual factors. Successful functioning is influenced, but is not solely dependent on, health condition or contextual factors (Talo & Rytökoski 2016). Thinking along the lines of the concept of functioning as described above means that the final judgment about how well or successful a person's functioning is must be primarily judged by the person themself.

Why use functioning as the focus for healthcare?

The concept of functioning in the context of health
One's individual functioning is a key component in health and wellbeing and requires direct consideration in healthcare systems (Madden et al. 2012). In the context of the modern conceptualisation of health as the 'ability to adapt and self-manage in the face of social, physical and emotional challenges' (Huber et al. 2011), functioning, characterised by ability/disability, can be understood as the operationalisation of health. This modern concept of health emphasises ability, adaptation and self-management in a biopsychosocial context. In accordance with its origins from the salutogenic approach (Antonovsky 1987, 1996), this is called 'positive health'. This can be seen as the counterpart of the biomedical pathogenic 'ill health' approach of current healthcare systems (Bengel et al. 1998, Huber et al. 2011). Both the salutogenic and the biopsychosocial perspectives point to the need to adopt, teach and systematically implement these into the future healthcare system as a whole (Adler 2009, Becker et al. 2010, Eriksson & Lindström 2005, Lezwijn et al. 2011, Sturmberg 2009, Zeyer 1997) (see Chapter 7). This will support the experience of 'being healthy', even though one's biological or physical capacities have become reduced by a 'health condition' (Tan et al. 2016). In other words, the operationalisation of the ICF concepts at the level of the individual are essentially personal, and emphasise that healthcare procedures, interventions and programs should reflect the idea of what human functioning is, and be developed in accordance with the physical, psychological, or social capacity and resources (capability), values and goals of the individual.

Functioning as a critical concept in healthcare
The WHO states:

> care inadequacies may result in patients being unable to maintain their 'functional ability', or lead to depression or early death. At best, health care is focused on meeting people's basic needs such as help with bathing or dressing, at the expense of broader objectives such as well-being and maintenance of dignity, personal choice and respect (WHO 2017).

This means that healthcare should be oriented towards optimising capacity and performance or compensating for lack of capacity so that functioning, as conceptualised in this chapter, is maintained and wellbeing more likely to be realised. Based on the principles of person-centred care, patients and their relatives have to be involved in care planning.

Functioning, as a focus for healthcare, thus asks for an approach focused on discovering the origins of health (salutogenesis) complementary to the pathogenic orientation focusing on the causes and precursors of disease.

How to work with the concept of functioning as a whole?

Functioning as the focus for healthcare requires a different healthcare system from our traditional disease-care approach. First, compared with disease-care, it is not possible to determine a general standard. In contrast with the concept of disease, this is the unique feature of the concept of functioning. To diagnose a disease, the health professional's focus is on the presence of specific, and mostly negative, indications to conclude that a person is experiencing a specific disease(s) or condition. Second, working in the concept of functioning means that initially the person themself comes up with aspects – abilities and challenges – relevant to their experienced functioning. The ICF can be used as a practical tool to operationalise the aspects of functioning. The framework of the ICF, used in its holistic biopsychosocial model, offers the opportunity to work with the patient's concept of functioning in a decision-making model.

Subsequently, the ICF terminology – 1 500 ICF categories – offers the opportunity to register, analyse and communicate about functioning. However, to describe one's functioning, it is impractical in terms of its size to use all the ICF categories. In principle, all the ICF categories are available and applicable to everyone. To describe one's individual status of functioning in a significant way the user themself chooses categories that are meaningfully related to a specific aim (Talo & Rytökoski 2016). Successful functioning obviously differs from person to person, and probably from one time to another in the life of the same person. What is necessary or meaningful in one personal situation may not work in another.

Last, but not least, the essence of working with the concept of functioning implies that the patient and their significant others are involved in making judgments and decisions about what is meaningful to them and therefore what issues, related to functioning, they want to address. Shared decision-making and person-centred care are key terms. This means that healthcare professionals sometimes have to accept that a patient can make a different choice related to their functioning – or their goals to achieve successful functioning – compared to what might be seen and judged as successful by healthcare professionals. In this way, the ICF represents an essentially 'democratic' 21st century approach to healthcare.

References

Adler RH (2009) Engel's biopsychosocial model is still relevant today. *J Psychosom Res* **67**(6): 607–611.

Antonovsky A (1987) *Unraveling the Mystery of Health. How People Manage Stress and Stay Well.* San Francisco CA: Jossey-Bass.

Antonovsky A (1996) The salutogenic model as a theory to guide health promotion. *Health Promotion International* **11**(1): 11–18.

Becker CM, Glascoff MA, Felts WM (2010) Salutogenesis 30 years later: Where do we go from here? Origins of Salutogenesis. *Int Elec J Health Ed* **13**: 25–32.

Bengel J, Strittmatter R, Willmann H (1998). *What keeps people healthy? The current state of discussion and the relevance of Antonvsky's salutogenetic model of health.* Germany: Federal Centre for Health Education (FCHE).

Bickenbach J (2014) Reconciling the capability approach and the ICF. *Alter* **8**: 10–23.

Bickenbach J, Cieza A, Rauch A, Stucki G (2012) *ICF Core Sets: Manual for Clinical Practice*, 1st edn. Göttingen Germany: Hogrefe Publishing.

Chou Y-C, Kröger T (2017) Application of the International Classification of Functioning Disability and Health in Taiwan victory of the medical model. *Disabil Soc* **32**(7): 1043–1064.

Engel GL (1977) The need for a new medical model: a challenge for biomedicine.*Science* **196**(4286): 129–136.

Eriksson M, Lindström B (2005) Validity of Antonovsky's sense of coherence scale: a systematic review. *J Epidemio Comm Health* **59**(6): 460–6.

Huber M, Knottnerus JA, Green L, et al. (2011) How should we define health? *BMJ* **343**: d4163.

Lezwijn J, Vaandrager L, Naaldenberg J, Wagemakers A, Koelen M, van Woerkum C (2011) Healthy ageing in a salutogenic way: building the HP 2.0 framework. *Health Soc Care Comm* **19**(1): 43–51.

Madden R, Ferreira M, Einfeld S, et al. (2012) New directions in health care and disability: the need for a shared understanding of human functioning. *Austr NZ J Pub Health* **36**(5): 458–461.

Sen A (1992) *Inequality Reexamined.* Oxford: Clarendon Press.

Stallinga HA (2015) *Human Functioning in Health Care. Application of the International Classification of Functioning Disability and Health (ICF).* Groningen: University of Groningen.

Sturmberg JP (2009) The personal nature of health. *J Eval Clin Pract* **15**(4): 749–754.

Talo SA, Rytökoski UM (2016) BPS-ICF model a tool to measure biopsychosocial functioning and disability within ICF concepts: theory and practice updated. *Int J Rehabil Res* **39**(1): 1–10.

Tan KK, Chan SWC, Wang W, Vehviläinen-Julkunen K (2016) A salutogenic program to enhance senseof coherence and quality of life for older people in the community: A feasibility randomized controlled trial and process evaluation. *Pat Ed Counsel* **99**(1): 108–116.

Wade DT, Halligan PW (2017) The biopsychosocial model of illness: a model whose time has come. *Clinic Rehab* **31**(8): 995–1004.

WHO (World Health Organization) (2001) *International Classification of Functioning Disability and Health: ICF.* Geneva: World Health Organization.

WHO (World Health Organization) (2017) *Towards long-term care systems in sub-Saharan Africa: WHO series on long-term care.* Geneva: World Health Organization.

Zeyer A (1997) Salutogenesis and pathogenesis – a change of paradigm viewed from the standpoint of modern physics. *Sozial-Und Präventivmedizin* **42**(6): 380–384.

Chapter 3

Personal factors in clinical practice and public health

Olaf Kraus de Camargo

The story of each of us is the story of an individual on the way to becoming a person. What makes us a person is not our ID card. The ID card has no room for those things that make us a person. What makes us a person is the way we think, the way we dream, the way we become others (Couto 2011).

Introduction

The WHO's International Classification of Functioning, Disability and Health (ICF) combines the biomedical model of health and the social model of health into a comprehensive biopsychosocial model (Fig. 3.1). The ICF recognises and documents psychological and contextual aspects of people's lives that, in addition to the biological characteristics of a person, are relevant – indeed essential – for health. As part of the 'contextual factors' (together with 'environmental' factors), the 'personal' factors of the ICF are defined as:

> the particular background of an individual's life and living and comprise features of the individual that are not part of their health condition or health states. These factors may include gender, race, age, other health conditions, fitness, lifestyle, habits, upbringing, coping styles, social background, education, profession, past and current experience (past life events and concurrent events), overall behaviour pattern and character style, individual psychological assets and other characteristics, all or any of which may play a role in disability at any level (WHO 2007).

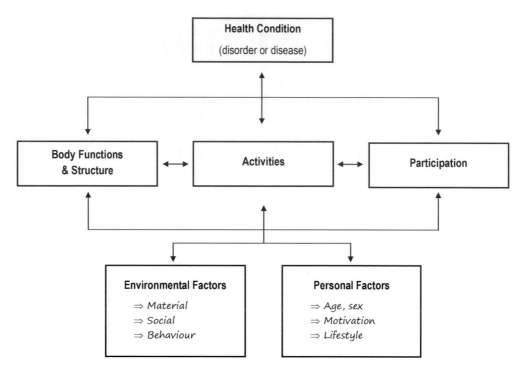

Figure 3.1 The ICF Framework with examples of environmental and personal contextual factors
Adapted from WHO 2001, p. 18, © 2001.

As noted in Chapter 1, a modern conceptualisation of health can be expressed as 'the ability to adapt and self-manage in the face of social, physical and emotional challenges' (Huber et al. 2011). In this way of thinking, functioning is characterised by ability and can be understood as the operationalisation of health. Extending this idea, according to the ICF, 'participation' refers to the involvement of a person in a life situation (one that is meaningful to them) without regard to how 'well' things are done. When describing functional health with the ICF information about the context of a person, it is essential that their personal factors are included. With the attempts over the last 15 years to use the ICF to describe the functioning status of populations, suggestions for defining and systematising personal factors have generated controversial discussions (Grotkamp et al. 2010, Ewert 2012, Simeonsson et al. 2014, Leonardi et al. 2015). The absence of defined categories and codes in the area of personal factors has been criticised, with the argument that without them the ICF only describes a person as a functioning object and there is a risk of losing sight of the person with his/her own values and characteristics (Duchan 2004). This concern, and the demand for defining personal factors more clearly and associate them with codes, is based on two fundamentally different usages of the ICF.

First, the ICF can be applied for individual care and support of people with different health conditions/disabilities/problems; and second, the ICF can be part of a larger population data collection to improve healthcare planning for populations or groups/cohorts with health problems. Attempts to define individual personal factors encounter the lack of a clear distinction regarding which observed aspects are inherent to a person and which are part of a specific situation that this person experiences during a certain moment. Some aspects could be part of the person's body structure or function and be coded accordingly under body functions and body structures, as for example, being unable to walk. On the other hand, the person might perceive exactly those aspects as unique factors that actually define them as a person (being a wheelchair user). The logic of the ICF (as with any classification) requires 'that single categories should be representing the intended concept clearly, precisely and unambiguously so that empirical conclusions can be made based on observable, testable or indirectly derived information' (WHO 2007). The following text further analyses and discusses the implications of this controversy.

Personal factors in the ICF

In considering the development of the ICF, from its test version, the ICIDH (International Classification of Impairments, Disabilities and Handicaps) (WHO 1980) (see Fig. 3.2), to the ICIDH-2, the main changes (and what we believe to be improvements) were the addition of 'contextual factors' (environmental factors and personal factors) and the adoption of a multidirectional framework rather than a linear model. The linear model in the ICIDH (WHO 1980) defined disability as a direct consequence of disease, and no aspects of the context were considered (Gray & Hendershot 2000).

To better understand the zeitgeist and compare the models that led to this development, it would be useful to refer to the publications of Badley, Nagi, Finkelstein, Chamie and Fougeyrollas (in Badley 1995). The group associated with Fougeyrollas in particular, defined personal factors as part of the body systems and abilities (Fougeyrollas et al. 2002, Levasseur et al. 2007). Based on the critiques of the ICIDH model (the lack of environmental factors and its linearity) (Thuriaux 1995), they developed the Disability Creation Process Model (DCP Model) (see Fig 3.3). In this model, the area of personal factors includes organic body systems as well as personal capabilities. This means that the components, body functions, structures, activities and personal factors of the ICF are all seen as being a part of the person. That person interacts with the environment to execute life habits. Under the influence of risk factors on the person, 'disability' is

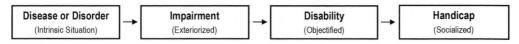

Figure 3.2 ICIDH Framework

Reprinted with permission from WHO 1980, p. 30.© 1980.

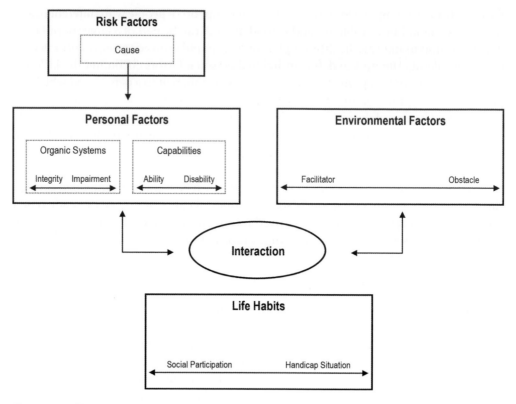

Figure 3.3 The Disability Creation Process
Adapted from Fougeyrollas et al. 1998, p. 166. © INDCP/CSICIDH 1998.

created through a change in that interaction – a change that is defined as the Disability Creation Process. Fougeyrollas et al. favour this model, with the argument that in order to decide about interventions it is relevant to know if those interventions will be directed towards the person or towards the environment, believing that each of these directions will require completely different approaches (Levasseur et al. 2007). Many aspects found in the DCP model under personal factors can also be found in the ICF in the components of body functions, structures and activities. Those attributions also depend on cultural and societal influences and can vary, as explained in the practical manual for the application of the ICF (WHO 2013). This is one of the reasons for the decision not to develop codes for elements of the personal factors.

Personal factors as the basis for treatment

Evidence-based medicine (EBM) is easily misunderstood as being simply the availability of scientific results derived from double-blind randomised studies. According to Guyatt, one of the leaders of evidence-based medicine, evidence-based practice refers to the convergence of three essential elements: the best available scientific evidence, the expertise and experience of the professional, coupled with the values and goals of the patient (Guyatt et al. 2008). Therefore, the expression of the personal aspects of the patient is an essential part of evidence-based practice and necessary for shared decision-making. EBM demands that professionals obtain relevant personal factors of their patients and consider these when making clinical decisions. Such an approach results in more individualised types of intervention. Patients included in a shared decision-making process achieve greater autonomy and empowerment (Institute of Medicine 2013). In clinical practice, it is therefore essential to capture personal factors and document them in order to understand, reduce or eliminate restrictions of participation. The question remains as to how best capture these personal factors and consider them when deciding about treatments.

What makes a person and how to describe them?

Even the origin of the term person describes something arbitrary and not transparent. The ancient Greeks used the term 'person' to refer to the masks used in Greek drama. Each mask was to symbolise a certain role that an actor played (Hoffe et al. 2002). Over time, the definition of the term person changed and moved from the ability to express one's own will, being rational, to being a synonym for a human being in different stages of development (consider, for example, the discussion of personhood in relation to early fetal diagnostics and abortion) (Hoffe et al. 2002). The philosopher Harry Frankfurt defines person as: 'those attributes which are the subject of our most humane concern with ourselves and the source of what we regard as most important and most problematical in our lives'. In this context, Frankfurt sees the essence of a person as closely related to the awareness of free will and their acting accordingly (Frankfurt 1971). Fox and Ward refer in their work to the philosophical publications of Deleuze and Guattari, who describe the subjectivity of a person as the result of a continuously changing 'assemblage' of a 'body without organs' with elements of the environment (Fox & Ward 2008). This concept was initially developed to understand the personality of people with schizophrenia. In comparison to the definition of Frankfurt they see the person not only as an acting subject but, depending on the situation, also understand the environment as part of that person.

In the field of rehabilitation Gibson et al. (2012) apply this concept in a case example summarised here: they present the girl Mimi in her environment. Depending on the situation, Mimi's identity changes. When she uses her wheelchair, she experiences herself with the wheelchair as one unit. In other situations, for example during body hygiene, she understands herself with her mother as one unit, and in other situations, for example during a conversation, she and her mother are both individual and separate persons, each part of the conversation with their own ideas and desires. This exemplifies that personal factors cannot be described with the same certainty or be organised into chapters as clinical findings that are related to the 'body with organs'. The categorisation and description of personal factors will always be subjective. To capture personal factors, it is essential to have the individual patient/client included in the process to understand their individual needs, their situation in life and their goals. Any decisions about therapy or rehabilitation to diminish restrictions of participation results from that interaction. In this perspective, and to allow the complete and individualised documentation of personal factors, the box for personal factors in the ICF framework is left empty. It can be understood as a blank sheet of paper to be filled collaboratively by patients and professionals according to the situation. Important personal factors can be documented in a narrative text instead of checking off pre-defined categories on a questionnaire.

The ICF and public health data

Physicians of the 19th century, including John Snow in England and Rudolf Virchow in Germany, recognised that the systematic collection of health and environmental data of a population is of fundamental importance for public health (Virchow 1848, Stanwell-Smith 2013). Based on their pioneering work, public health services were established around the world and the role of the state as a responsible and active player in the maintenance of population health was established (Fee & Brown 2005). After these first revolutionary developments, the systematic collection of health data has become a standard. The classification systems of the World Health Organization are valuable instruments in those efforts at standardisation. The launch of the ICF was linked to the hope of obtaining a better understanding of the health situation of populations than that which classic health statistics alone could deliver. In addition to information about diagnoses, immunisation rates and mortality rates it was hoped to obtain relevant information concerning the social aspects of disease and disability. Wenzel and Morfeld describe an increased use of the ICF in different areas of action starting from Early Intervention services to Workplace Rehabilitation (Wenzel & Morfeld 2015). They also describe international examples of the ICF being used to define indicators of health and a better assessment of barriers and facilitators to improve the inclusion of people with disabilities. In Germany, the ICF is mentioned in the public health report but the systematic capture of ICF data has not yet been established.

With current rapid technological developments, it is probable that the individual challenges of citizens with health problems will be captured in different ways than how traditional health statistics have been collected. Instead of centralised surveys being sent through institutions and administrators of healthcare systems, it is now possible for citizens to capture and share their data independently (http://www.myhealthmydata.eu). People become the owners, administrators and transmitters of data. The first examples for such initiatives can be found in Finland where electronic health portals are being developed to collect ICF-based data shared by the citizens (Antilla 2016). Such a development allows a real-time analysis of the health situation of the population and can contribute to improved functional health and social participation of citizens independent of purely medical diagnostic criteria. In addition, such initiatives allow us to capture contextual factors such as the social and physical environment of the population, which then can inform the need for regulations and policies with the goal of improving general wellbeing. Citizens can use the technology to share their functional status proactively instead of waiting for surveys to be sent to them or being part of a selected group of a single institution or department. This initiative is part of the political decision that has been made in Finland to combine the services from the ministries of social welfare and health into one ministry, which reflects the current understanding of health within a biopsychosocial model (Ministry of Social Affairs and Health – Finland 2012).

Personal factors and public health

The goal of capturing population-level data is to be able to aggregate and analyse these data and make them available for political decisions. From a biomedical perspective, the fight against diseases requires data about causal agents such as toxins and pathogens. As mentioned previously, as early as in the 19th century John Snow and Robert Virchow stated that data about the environment (e.g. contaminated water wells, poverty, famine) are equally important to improve population health.

Today, we are able to describe the environment using ICF data and can therefore capture not only physical contextual factors but also factors such as the availability of assistive devices, health personnel, teachers and the attitudes of these professionals and other members of the community towards people with chronic health conditions and disabilities. These are additional valuable insights that will possibly not only allow further physical changes to eliminate barriers in our environment, but also inform new policies and laws to improve participation, reduce barriers in all areas of public life, thus strengthening the position of people with chronic health conditions and disabilities in our society. In contrast to the situation in the 19th century, in many countries today population health is not about the survival of people threatened by infections but about the coexistence and equal participation of people of all abilities and limitations in a diverse society.

What role could the systematic capture of personal factors have within such a vision? Geyh et al. (2011) provide a literature review of the use of personal factors and propose a list of candidates for such a classification. Another group of German-speaking professionals, initiated by the MDK (Medizinischer Dienst Niedersachsen, a medical advisory for insurance companies) from Lower Saxony published a consensus paper with an even more detailed list of categories for personal factors associated with alphanumeric codes (Grotkamp et al. 2010, 2012, 2014). According to the authors the goal of their proposal is to allow for more transparency and reproducible decisions when services for rehabilitation are being granted within the German system. They hope that such a process contributes in such a way that 'the results are not randomly dependent on which person is assessing the patient'. The fact that body functions could also be understood as a personal factor is being addressed in their proposal by defining any normal body function as a personal factor. Such a procedure omits the situation that some people with specific diagnoses might identify exactly with their body functions or structures that are different from the norm, as they feel that those differences characterise them as a person and are part of their identity, even if different from typical. Theoretically, this could lead to a classificatory dilemma where categories that are deviant from the norm would be coded both as personal factors and body functions. This runs against the required clarity and avoidance of ambiguity necessary for any classification system. It is also a step back in time, focusing on normalisation (ableism) instead of functioning and participation.

An attempt to use personal factors in a practical setting was published by Geyh et al. (2016). They describe the psychological personal factors of patients with spinal cord injuries. This carefully developed study enriches the discussion about the practicability and utility of defining personal factors (Geyh et al. 2016). Different instruments of personality diagnostics, coping mechanisms and quality of life were used. Over 500 patients were surveyed about their feelings, thoughts, beliefs, coping processes and quality of life. The analysis, carried out using different variants and groups, showed that most patients presented a relatively limited negative affect and a moderate positive affect. The majority interpreted difficult life situations not as a loss or a threat, but as a positive challenge. In general, the patients were satisfied with their life situations and presented good social competencies and problem-solving abilities (Geyh et al. 2016). The study presents a positive overall situation of these study patients, possibly related to the quality of the treatment received as well as people's capacity to adapt to new situations and new personal realities. Both groups, i.e. Grotkamp et al. and Geyh et al., argue that the documentation of personal factors adds important additional information about the patients. While the methodology of Grotkamp et al. to reach a consensus can be criticised (being too professionally-focused and not including a variety of patient perspectives) (Ewert 2012), Geyh et al. present a useful approach to the discussion by collecting actual patient data. Building on that approach, they present a way to describe and define personal factors by conceptualising them as the full range of features of a person in terms of 'individual facts, immediate subjective experience, and recurrent patterns of experience and behaviour' (Geyh et al. 2018).

The question arises, though, whether the categories and findings reported by Geyh et al. do in fact represent the relevant personal factors that patients would choose on their own to describe themselves and their life situations. How is it possible to conclude from results of a series of questionnaires that those answers describe 'the specific life situation of each individual' and are 'not part of their health problem' (see p. 25)?

Would the patients of the study make exactly those statements about their own coping abilities, their beliefs and feelings if they were asked to describe themselves as a person? Would they feel that these factors were important for the decisions about their treatments? And, would they agree that those factors are having an important influence on their participation?

The information collected in the questionnaires certainly is important and helpful. But it does not make the case that we require the definition of single categories with codes to describe personal factors to obtain that type of information.

The risks of capturing personal factors

The collection and transmission of personal factors for deciding about the access to health services creates several difficulties and risks. On the level of the ICF, the creation of defined categories for personal factors would preclude the ability to separate them from other domains of functioning, as this is a personal decision. In addition, the coding of categories with qualifiers would lead to the creation of a scale of values regarding personal factors. The result would be that the ICF would be transformed from a classification of functional health towards a classification of persons, which is explicitly *not* the purpose of the ICF (WHO 2013). On the level of interpersonal relations, the introduction of values (qualifiers) of personal factors can lead to undesired consequences. Any time we establish a relationship with another person, we evaluate each other; this also happens within the physician–patient relationship. Each one creates a picture with values of each other. This evaluation modulates the interaction, but it is not explicitly expressed or documented and only will be mentioned if it is important for the therapeutic process (for example, the observed pattern of coming late to appointments can be addressed within a consultation or a therapeutic relationship, but should not drive the decision to grant services or not). When an exposure of personal aspects is necessary, it occurs within the protective space of the clinician–patient relationship. When, on the other hand, personal aspects start to be coded, evaluated and transmitted in a patient chart (to justify decisions made about the access to care), there might be dangerous consequences. Besides leading to a potential discrimination of patients based on their personal characteristics and valuations by health professionals, patients might internalise such evaluations made within a power-based relationship, with additional detrimental effects. Over 60 years ago, Bertram Forer demonstrated how easily so-called individualised assessments were accepted as true and valid by students who had all received the exact same wording as part of their 'personality' assessment (Forer 1949). The systematic capturing of personal factors is therefore no guarantee for transparency and traceability. It can cause unintended harm and result in a higher risk of discrimination without adding value for public health. Based on all these considerations, the authors of this book fully support the current approach of the ICF not to codify 'personal factors'.

Conclusion

The ICF is an excellent tool for improving our understanding of health and disability. It can be used to develop functional profiles containing more meaningful information than it is possible to obtain from a list of diagnoses. Professionals need to be aware of, and get to know, the personal factors of their patients to better understand their values, desires and goals. This is considered essential for evidence-based practice.

The collection and documentation of personal factors should be reserved to the personal interaction between the people that are part of the circle of care. Personal factors cannot be defined and coded for statistical purposes, as the necessary categories do not correspond to the individual variations of how people define themselves. For statistical purposes, other instruments, tools and classifications can be used to complement some of the aspects not found in the ICF (WHO 2013, Leonardi et al. 2015).

References

Antilla H (2016) Feasibility study of a patient-driven mobile ICF-based assessment tool (mICF) [online]. *icfmobile.org*. http://icfmobile.org/2016/01/29/hello-world/.

Badley EM (1995) The genesis of handicap: definition models of disablement and role of external factors. *Disabil Rehabil* **17**: 53–62.

Couto M (2011) *E se Obama Fosse Africano?* Sao Paulo: Companhia das Letras.

Duchan JF (2004) Where is the person in the ICF? *Adv Speech Lang Path* **6**(1): 63–65.

Ewert T (2012) Stellungnahme der DGRW zu 'Personbezogene Faktoren der ICF – Entwurf der AG "ICF" des Fachbereichs II der Deutschen Gesellschaft für Sozialmedizin und Prävention (DGSMP)'. *Die Rehabilitation* **51**(2): 129–130.

Fee E, Brown TM (2005) The Public Health Act of 1848. *Bull World Health Organ* **83**(11): 866–867.

Forer BR (1949) The fallacy of personal validation: A classroom demonstration of gullibility. *J Abnorm Psychol* **44**(1): 118–123.

Fougeyrollas P, Cloutier R, Bergeron H, Côté J, St Michel G (1998) *The Québec Classification Disability Creation Process*. Québec: International Network on Disability Creation Process (INDCP)/CSICIDH.

Fougeyrollas P, Noreau L, Boschen KA (2002) Interaction of environment with individual characteristics and social participation: Theoretical perspectives and applications in persons with spinal cord injury. *Top Spinal Cord Inj Rehabil* **7**(3): 1–16.

Fox NJ, Ward KJ (2008) What are health identities and how may we study them? *Sociol Health Illness* **30**(7): 1007–1021.

Frankfurt HG (1971) Freedom of the will and the concept of a person. *J Philosoph* **68**(1): 5–20.

Geyh S, Peter C, Muller R, et al. (2011) The personal factors of the International Classification of Functioning Disability and Health in the literature – a systematic review and content analysis. *Disabil Rehabil* **33**(13–14): 1089–1102.

Geyh S, Kunz S, Müller R, Peter C (2016) Original report describing functioning and health after spinal cord injury in the light of psychological – personal factors for the SwiSCI Study Group. *J Rehabil Med* **48**: 219–234.

Geyh S, Schwegler U, Peter C, Müller R (2018) Representing and organizing information to describe the lived experience of health from a personal factors perspective in the light of the International Classification of Functioning, Disability and Health (ICF): a discussion paper. *Disabil Rehabil* 1–12.

Gibson BE, Carnevale FA, King G (2012) 'This is my way': reimagining disability in/dependence and interconnectedness of persons and assistive technologies. *Disabil Rehabil* **34**(22): 1894–1899.

Gray DB, Hendershot GE (2000) The ICIDH-2: Developments for a new era of outcomes research. *Arch Physical Med Rehabil* **81**(12)Suppl2: 10–14.

Grotkamp S, Cibis W, Behrens J, et al. (2010) Personbezogene Faktoren der ICF – Entwurf der AG 'ICF' des Fachbereichs II der Deutschen Gesellschaft für Sozialmedizin und Prävention [Personal contextual factors of the ICF draft from the Working Group 'ICF' of Specialty Group II of the German Society for Social Medicine and Prevention]. *Gesundheitswesen* **72**(12): 908–916.

Grotkamp S, Cibis W, Nuchtern E, Baldus A, Behrens J, Bucher PO, et al. (2012) [Personal factors of the ICF]. *Gesundheitswesen* **74**(7): 449–458.

Grotkamp S, Cibis W, Bahemann A, Baldus A, Behrens J, Nyffeler ID, et al. (2014) Bedeutung der personbezogenen Faktoren der ICF für die Nutzung in der praktischen Sozialmedizin und Rehabilitation [Relevance of personal contextual factors of the ICF for use in practical social medicine and rehabilitation]. *Gesundheitswesen* **76**: 172–180.

Guyatt G, Rennie D, Meade MO, Cook DJ (2008) *JAMA's Users's Guide to the Medical Literature: A Manual for Evidence-Based Clinical Practice*, 2nd edn. New York: McGraw-Hill.

Hoffe O, Forschner M, Horn C, Vossenkuhl W (eds.) (2002) Person. In: Höffe O, *Lexikon der Ethik*. München: Verlag CH. Beck oHG, pp. 198–200.

Huber M, Knottnerus JA, Green L, van der Horst H, Jadad AR, Kromhout D, et al. (2011) How should we define health? *BMJ* **343**: d4163.

Institute of Medicine IOM (2013) *Partnering with Patients to Drive Shared Decisions Better Value and Care Improvement: Workshop Proceedings*. Washington, DC: The National Academies Press.

Leonardi M, Sykes C, Madden RC, et al. (2015) Do we really need to open a classification box on personal factors in ICF? *Disabil Rehabil* **38**(13):1327–1328.

Levasseur M, Desrosiers J and St-Cyr Tribble D (2007) Comparing the Disability Creation Process and International Classification of Functioning Disability and Health Models. *Can J Occ Ther* **74**(ICF Special Issue): 233–242.

Ministry of Social Affairs and Health – Finland (2012) National Development Programme for Social Welfare and Health Care (Kaste). http://stm.fi/en/kaste-progamme.

Simeonsson RJ, Lollar D, Bjorck-Akesson E, et al. (2014) ICF and ICF-CY lessons learned: Pandora's box of personal factors. *Disabil Rehabil* **36**(25): 2187–2194.

Stanwell-Smith R (2013) The remarkable Dr John Snow. *Perspect Pub Health* **133**(5): 237.

Thuriaux MC (1995) The ICIDH: evolution status and prospects. *Disabil Rehabil* **17**(3–4): 112–118.

Virchow RC (1848) *Mittheilungen über die in Oberschlesien herrschende Typhus-Epidemie*. Archiv für path Anat u Physiol u fur klin Medicin. Berlin: G. Reimer.

Wenzel T, Morfeld M (2015) Die Internationale Klassifikation der Funktionsfähigkeit Behinderung und Gesundheit (ICF) – Eine Expertise im Auftrag der Deutschen Gesellschaft für Rehabilitationswissenschaften e.V. (DGRW e.V.). [*The International Classification of Functioning, Disability and Health – Expert Report for the German Society for Rehabilitation Sciences*]. Stendal: German Society for Rehabilitation Sciences. http://dgrw-online.de/files/icf_expertise_dgrw_homepage.pdf.

WHO (World Health Organization) (1980) *International Classification of Impairments Disabilities and Handicaps*. Geneva: World Health Organization.

WHO (World Health Organization) (2001) *International Classification of Functioning Disability and Health: ICF*. Geneva: World Health Organization.

WHO (World Health Organization) (2007) *International Classification of Functioning Disability and Health – Children and Youth Version, 1st edn*. Geneva: World Health Organization.

WHO (World Health Organization) (2013) *How to use the ICF: A practical manual for using the International Classification of Functioning Disability and Health (ICF). Exposure draft for comment*. Geneva: World Health Organization.

Chapter 4

Marriage between the ICF and patient-reported outcome measures (PROMS): How good is the relationship?

Gabriel M Ronen

Scenario

Cassandra M is a medical professional involved in providing care for children and young adults with neurodevelopmental conditions in a medium-sized town's health community centre. She is also a member of a professional organisation that endorses the introduction and routine use of the World Health Organization's (WHO) International Classification of Functioning, Disability and Health (ICF). Cassandra recognises the potential benefits of this framework for her own institution, as well as her patients and their families. She also acknowledges the value of patient- or person-reported outcomes in evaluating the programs and services at the centre from her clients' own perspectives. She introduced her colleagues to the ICF framework and the idea of linking the ICF with person-reported outcome measures. She focused primarily on addressing the following question: How can our interventions improve the functioning of young people in the face of chronic impairments – from their own perspectives?

The resistance of some of her co-workers to adopt these novel concepts surprised Cassandra. She offered to follow up with weekly discussions with the intention to listen to and understand her fellow professionals' questions and concerns. She quickly realised that some of her co-workers raised important questions for which she was unprepared, nor had she any evidence-based answers ready at hand. She also realised that answering some of the questions deserved a thorough review of the scientific literature. Cassandra listed the following questions that she felt needed further exploration and took a brief sabbatical leave to study the issues raised by her co-workers. This elaborate process felt like delving into uncharted waters. Her questions included:

- *What is meant by health and patient-reported outcomes within the context of the ICF framework?*

- *Do patients share my views on whether an intervention generates more good than harm?*

- *What is the best way to find out whether patients have additional or different concerns about their health and functioning?*

- *What sort of knowledge do I need prior to selecting patient-reported outcome measures (PROMs)?*

- *What is the rationale for the routine use of PROMs?*

- *How can I find out the intended purpose of a PROM?*

- *Will the self-reported measures capture the expected outcomes of the patient following an intervention?*

- *Who would be the best person to complete the PROM questionnaire?*

- *Are there any specific ethical implications for using PROMs in children?*

- *Are there any practical tips to facilitate the use of PROMs in my practice?*

Introduction

The ICF and PROMs are two distinct and unrelated entities. The ICF framework describes health through the lens of functioning, as discussed in the introduction to this book and in related chapters (see especially Chapter 2). This current chapter discusses the potential opportunities regarding whether and how one can involve individual patients or populations in evaluating and measuring – from their perspectives – the successes and failures of programs, services and interventions that use and rely on the ICF framework and related constructs. The author of this chapter, and many others in the field, believe that it should be possible for individuals with health concerns and impairments to report on their own health, functioning and capabilities as viewed from their own perspectives, expectations, values and goals, and in so doing, take part in modifying and hopefully improving the continuum of care.

This chapter explains what person (patient)-reported outcomes (PROs) are and explores why individuals or their surrogate proxies are well-situated to evaluate their own health, functioning and quality of life, and in so doing become active participants in their own healthcare decisions when they wish to do so. Linking all these concepts makes sense ethically, as it promotes patients' autonomy (for those who wish to participate in decision-making); focuses on interventions that improve self-defined functioning rather than just biomedical markers; and therefore strives to generate outcomes that do more good than harm as judged by the people receiving the services. This linkage also seems fair and just for both the individuals and their close social network within the context of their environment and self-defined goals.

In addition, the author will try to answer Cassandra's questions, focusing on PROMs, and will illustrate how one may want to integrate and use these concepts in daily practice.

Basic concepts

What is health?

This seemingly simple question may mean different things to different people. The ICF views health as a dynamic process among the interconnected categories of functioning and contextual factors. In the setting of this book the author believes that the definition of health needs to reflect the ICF framework and focus on what people can do or want to do, and support them to be able to follow and achieve their goals and expectations. This concept embraces the idea that any person who can achieve their goals would be considered as potentially healthy irrespective of any impairment of body structure or function. Accordingly, Huber et al. (2011) proposed to define positive health as: 'the ability to adapt and to self-manage, in the face of social, physical and emotional challenges'. Consequently, achieving health would not depend on achieving the utopian desire for perfect physical, cognitive and social status as defined in 1948 for the constitution of the World Health Organization (United Nations 1948). This distinction between the realistic and utopian concepts of health is particularly important when we come to think about population data such as those from the Centers for Disease Control and Prevention (2015) to remind us that approximately one in five adults in the US reports some type of disability ('impairment' in ICF terminology). From the humanistic and psychosocial perspectives, persons with impairments should never be considered, a priori, as having poor health or being disabled.

In a mixed-methods quantitative and qualitative study with stakeholders from the Netherlands, Huber and colleagues identified six dimensions for their broad concept of 'positive health', namely: (1) bodily functions, (2) cognitive functions and perceptions, (3) spiritual dimension, (4) quality of life, (5) social and societal participation and (6) daily functioning (Huber et al. 2016). A systematic review revealed that the spiritual dimension is also an important coping strategy for children with health conditions (Reynolds et al. 2016). Not surprisingly, most patients preferred to have all of these dimensions assessed, in contrast to physicians and policy makers who

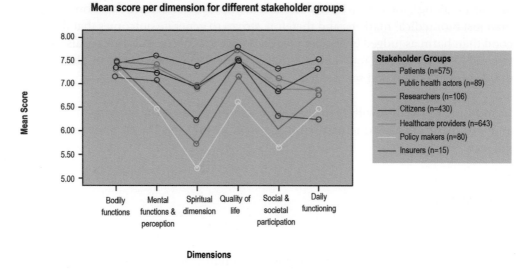

Figure 4.1 Mean scores per stakeholder group on a nine-point scale, indicating the importance assigned by respondents to a dimension as being part of 'health'

Reproduced from Huber et al. 2016, with permission from BMJ Publishing Group Ltd.

preferred to evaluate health more narrowly, and who limited their concerns to its biomedical interpretation. However, for physicians who had themselves experienced a chronic disease, the spiritual/existential dimension and social and societal participation became more important than for their co-professionals (Figure 4.1) (Huber et al. 2016). As we see, this recent broad definition is built upon and expands the ICF concept of health. It will become apparent that most PROMs lag significantly behind in evaluating all these dimensions.

What are health outcomes?

There are different conceptualisations as to what health outcomes represent. The following definition fits well into the perspectives of the ICF theory:

> Health outcomes can *therefore* be thought of as changes in the global health or any of its core dimensions of an individual, group or population, attributable to a planned intervention or series of interventions regardless of whether such an intervention was intended to cause any change (adapted from definition of health outcomes Mayo 2015 p. 680).

The term *outcome* should be kept separate from the term *prognosis,* which we regard as the expected end point of the natural trajectory of a disease or condition (Ronen & Rosenbaum 2013 p. 12).

What are person- or patient-reported outcomes (PROs)?

PRO is a contemporary umbrella term for any aspect of a personal report of an individual's health that comes directly from that person (including children and caregivers). These reports reflect the person's life experience and values, in relation to their health condition and its management, without the interpretation of these persons' responses by healthcare professionals or others. We prefer to use the term 'person' rather than 'patient' to describe PROs because traditionally it is widely believed that there are more dimensions to a person's life than are considered when we only think about the person in the role of patient, usually characterised in relation to the healthcare system in the context of a disease, condition or impairment. PROs are today considered the criterion standard to evaluate patients, even if they are children, and they play an important role in person- and family-centred healthcare (Ronen 2016).

The term PRO was created to meet the need for developing a terminology upon which healthcare providers and policy makers could agree. This term was chosen to move away from the unsettling confusion created by the different conceptualisations of the terms health-related quality of life (HRQoL) and Quality of Life (QoL) that resulted in lack of equivalence and comparability among measures titled by the term HRQoL or QoL, and imposed a barrier for communication and research in this field (Wallander & Koot 2016). The term PRO overcomes these conceptual problems by focusing on the source of information and by emphasising the importance of the individual's own perspectives when coming to decide about potential interventions and management (Valderas & Alonso 2008).

Why do we need to measure different aspects of health?

Stucki and colleagues (2008) stressed that 'if we aim towards a comprehensive understanding of human functioning (and other aspects of health), and the development of comprehensive programs to optimise functioning (and health) of individuals and populations we need to develop suitable measures' (p. 315). These authors believe that the development of the universal ICF model marked 'an important step in the development of measurement instruments and ultimately for our understanding of functioning, disability and health' (pp. 315–6). Obviously, we need to expand this contention to all aspects of health that can be reported by affected individuals, groups and populations.

Routine measurement of functioning and other aspects of health will give us the necessary feedback on the usefulness of our services, programs and interventions as judged by the people receiving those services. This kind of evidence will aid government and funding agencies in deciding which services should remain, expand or close down (Duncan & Murray 2012).

What are PROMs and why do we need them?

PROMs explicitly refer to standardised and validated person – (patient-) reported out-come measures (including any self-reported scales or items) that cannot be captured directly through other means (Dawson et al. 2010). PROMs were originally developed, in part, to aid in evaluating and comparing effectiveness of healthcare interventions (Black et al. 2016). Healthcare providers can use PROMs to focus on a person's individual health goals and guide diagnostic and management decisions. Through PROMs, healthcare providers and policy makers can learn whether patients share our professional perspectives about their health and wellbeing, whether they have additional or different concerns, and what those are. PROMs can teach us whether our patients are truly better after interventions by following the ethical principle of doing more good than harm (Beauchamp & Childress 2013) within the context of their own life. Importantly, PROMs help us evaluate a variety of health-related constructs and the changes in trajectories over time and in relation to what we recommend. So far, most generic PROMs do not cover all the broad areas of life identified by Huber and colleagues (Huber et al. 2016). These latter researchers suggested a potential model for each person's self-reported outcome profile at any point in time (see Figure 4.2).

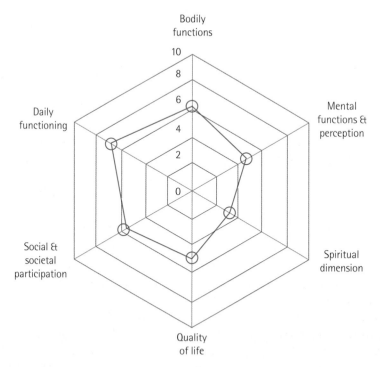

Figure 4.2 The six dimensions on a subjective scale, visualised for practical use, indicating a fictional estimation of a person's state of 'positive health'

Reproduced from Huber et al. 2016, with permission from BMJ Publishing Group Ltd.

This model incorporates the ICF components but specifies additional dimensions that are concealed within the contextual boxes of the ICF model. PROMs are additionally used to monitor quality and performance in health systems. Fortunately, important advances have been made in communicating PROMs with the international consensus on taxonomy, terminology and definitions of measurement properties for PROMs that should help interested healthcare providers and policy makers better understand the content of PROM publications (Mokkink et al. 2010).

In this illustrated (Figure 4.2) fictional personal account of daily functioning, body functions and participation were reported as moderate; mental health and QoL were somewhat worse and the spiritual dimension was the poorest scored dimension. This scale would help the clinician to focus on the poorest patient-reported domains by consulting, with the patient's permission, their chosen spiritual leader to help identify the underlying issues and work with the patient towards a potential resolution.

Theoretical considerations linking PROMs and the ICF

Can we integrate PROMs into the ICF classification model?
Valderas and Alonso (2008) indicated that 'classification and evaluation systems (like the ICF and PROMs) are complementary and should be used in tandem' (p. 1 131). These authors have developed an integrated conceptual model, built on an earlier biopsychosocial model by Wilson and Cleary (1995) and enhanced by identifying a minimal set of consistent concepts incorporated into the ICF framework (Figure 4.3). This multifaceted model allows the classification of most measurement instruments and is designed to facilitate 'a more adequate selection and application of these instruments' (p. 1 125). The main guiding concepts for this classification are (1) the construct or the measurement objective, (2) the population (i.e. age, sex, condition or culture) and (3) the measurement model (see Valderas & Alonso 2008 for details). Another useful benchmark for such a classification would be to include the purpose and intended use of the instrument. Importantly, any classification system linked to a conceptual framework would meaningfully help identify a pool of PROMs for any given purpose. In their model the authors differentiate and define the concepts that apply to PROMs, consisting of (1) symptom status, (2) functional status, (3) health perception, and (4) overall QoL (the latter conceptualised as subjective wellbeing). Obviously, the biological and physiological domains do not lend themselves to PROs. These authors also implied the need to consider satisfaction with the healthcare provision and resilience as additional important PRO constructs. Within the classification system these latter constructs can be included in the contextual factors of the ICF.

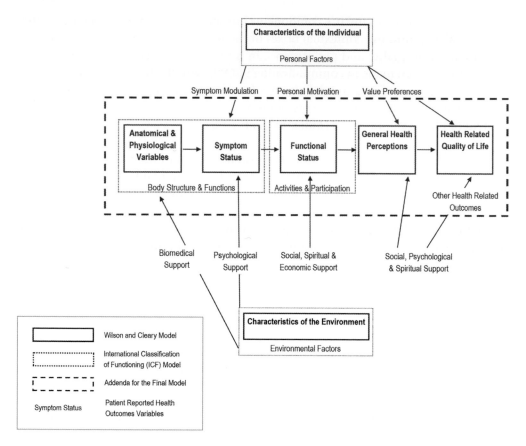

Figure 4.3 An integrated descriptive model of health outcomes
Reprinted by permission from Valderas & Alonso 2008. © 2008.

Routine data collections

At the conceptual level, prospective longitudinal data collection is essential; such data enable us to recognise the trajectories of health, functioning, quality of life and other contextual constructs, and in turn allowing us to understand more fully the natural history of populations with various conditions and people's own evaluations of our recommended interventions to illustrate trajectory classes of quality of life in children with epilepsy (Ferro et al. 2017). Electronic and paper form data will allow the practicing clinician to follow each patient's profile longitudinally. The process can be significantly enhanced once the health provider reviews the questionnaire results with the patient. Such individual involvement would also help maintain the long-term trust relationships between patients and clinicians. The routine use of PROMs may also increase the frequency of discussion of patient outcomes during the clinic visit (Kotronoulas et al. 2014). It seems that patients tend to accept the more efficient electronic data collections if these systems serve their needs.

As mentioned earlier, PROMs need to be completed by the persons themselves, even if they are children or individuals with cognitive impairments. Assistance with questionnaires should not come directly from the caregivers or members of the clinical team. However, proxy respondents may be needed to complete PROMs when the patients themselves are unable to do so.

PROMs: Moving from theory and research to mainstream clinical practice

Meaningful application of PROMs in ICF-oriented practices
As described above, research has provided us with ample evidence that at the conceptual level the ICF and PROMs complement and enhance each other as a seemingly perfect match. Now we need to examine whether this marriage can fit into our daily practice routine.

At both the conceptual and practical level PROMS are usually divided into generic and condition-specific measures. Examples for generic PROMs in use in child health are the European-developed KIDSCREEN and the US-developed PedQL® measures. Both measures allow children, and separately their caregivers, to complete the questionnaires. However, although both have been labelled as quality of life measures, they differ in a number of essential aspects that may not be apparent to the practicing clinician (see Table 4.1). Condition-specific measures, on the other hand, assess particular aspects or dimensions of the health of individuals with similar underlying biomedical conditions. These include health functioning, symptoms, quality of life or other dimensions. Similar to generic measures, several condition-specific PROMs, such as those for cerebral palsy and epilepsy, vary in specific aspects of their content and may not be interchangeable (Sadeghi et al. 2014, Schiariti et al. 2014). Likewise, instruments for participation also vary in the proportion and number of participation domains they include (Chien et al. 2014).

In practice, it becomes intimidating to realise that there are several thousand PROMs available, and new ones are developed every day (Quality of Life Instruments Database – PROQOLID) (eProvide 2002). Some of these measures were developed prior to the ICF publication and therefore lack any reference to its framework. The following sections focus on how clinicians can choose PROMs.

Can we use the ICF as a framework to analyse the content of PROMs?
The ICF has been used in multiple studies to provide a standardised framework to outline the health content found in measures (e.g. Cieza & Stucki 2005, Fayed et al. 2012, Janssens et al. 2015). First, these authors used the WHO definitions to distinguish the

Table 4.1   Generic patient-reported child and adolescent outcome measures: conceptual content using WHO definitions

Instrument name	Dominant perspective	Dominant ICF components	Instrument summary
Child Health and Illness Profile	FDH with an unknown subcomponent	Body functions and activity and participation	FDH instrument
Child Health Questionnaire	FDH with QoL and unknown features	Activities and participation	FDH with some QoL features
DISABKIDs	QoL with some functioning features	Body functions, activities and participation and environment	QoL instrument with biopsychosocial components
KIDSCREEN	QoL with some functioning features	Activities and participation	QoL with biopsychosocial components
PedsQL 4.0	FDH	Activities and participation	FDH instrument
Health Utility Index	FDH with one QoL attribute	Body functions	FDH instrument with emphasis on body functions
Satisfaction with Life Scale (Diener)	QoL	None	QoL instrument

ICF: International Classification of Functioning Disability and Health; FDH: functioning, disability and health; QoL – quality of life.

Adapted from Fayed et al. 2012.

biopsychosocial and spiritual health from HRQoL/QoL approaches found in multidimensional PRO instruments. Second, they described the health content within each of the instruments by coding them within the framework of the ICF. Using the ICF, these and related studies also described the health content of the PROMs more explicitly. The multidimensional nature of health as outlined by the WHO within the ICF implies that PROMs of functioning should cover a mix of body functions, activities and participation, environmental, and personal factors to represent a *balanced* biopsychosocial and spiritual health perspective. At present, most PROMS exclude at least one major ICF domain and conflate aspects of functioning and wellbeing (Janssens et al. 2015). These ideas are illustrated in Table 4.1, in which a selection of child and adolescent measures are reviewed.

What other aspects need consideration when choosing PROMs?
Beyond strong psychometric properties (Streiner et al. 2015) any measure needs to be evaluated by the intended population (meaning those with either the same condition or symptoms). In addition, one should identify whether the content of the measure was identified by a sample of the population of interest, which is usually achieved through well-defined and hopefully robust qualitative methodologies.

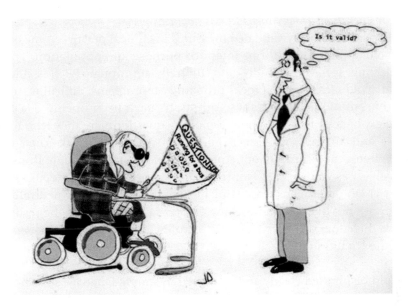

Figure 4.4 Existing PROMs may include questions irrelevant to the population of interest
Reproduced from Dawson et al. 2010, with permission from BMJ Publishing Group Ltd.

In recent years, researchers have elaborated on what to look for when choosing a PROM (Waters et al. 2009, Fayed 2013). Moreover, existing PROMs may include questions irrelevant to the population of interest (Figure 4.4). For this and other reasons the Patient-Reported Outcome Measurement Information System (PROMIS) provides item banks for measuring PROs for a variety of conditions and populations (Riley et al. 2010). Item banks allow people to select customised short scales that can easily be used longitudinally, or can be administered in a sequence and length determined by a computer programmed for precision and clinical relevance.

Data collection approaches that support and streamline the use of PROMs in our individual daily healthcare practices are still significantly underdeveloped, and health policy recommendations have not yet demonstrated the practicality of integrating PROMs into clinical practice (Van der Wees et al. 2014). To date, only the NHS program in the UK has shown evidence that large scale systematic PROMs collection is feasible. Hutchings and colleagues (2012) identified the subpopulations that were less likely to respond to pre- and post-operative PROM questionnaires in a trial of 131,447 individuals who underwent elective surgery. Examples included patients in the most deprived quintile for socio-economic status, patients who had poorer pre-operative health, and those who had been assisted when completing their pre-operative questionnaire (Hutchings et al. 2012). This study highlights the possibility of responder bias that needs to be taken into consideration when interpreting population PROMs results. For example, people with poorer health status, who are in a particular age range or a socio-economic group may differ in their response patterns from other subgroups.

Practical considerations concerning PROMs applications
It is unethical to use poorly validated measures in clinical practice. A measure needs to be selected appropriately for its intended purpose and population. This should include selecting: age-, vulnerability- and culturally-appropriate PROMs. Additionally, one should avoid measures that focus primarily on problems, difficulties, challenges and negative emotions. Unless these questions have been openly discussed and their value explained prior to completion of the questionnaire they tend to threaten both adults' and children's self-esteem and endorse negative self-concepts. Examples of negative items that illustrate our concern include: (1) Do people think that you are not as clever as you are? (2) Is it frustrating to be unable to keep up with other children? (3) Do other teens tease you? Ideally, items should be neutrally phrased so that they are not likely to impose any emotional burden, lead the respondent in an expected direction, or, indeed, portray a professional's assumptions regarding the impact of the condition.

Items should be phrased clearly and expressed in simple language so as not to cause any cognitive burden. For example, is it ethical to exclude subpopulations with cognitive impairments from responding to PROMs? Avoid any acronyms like 'PedsQL' or 'PROMIS'. Furthermore, explain that there are no right or wrong answers, and allow provisions for responses like 'I'm not really sure' or 'I don't know'.

One may argue correctly that all PROMs need to be valid for the respondents asked to use them (as illustrated in Figure 4.4). However, there appears to be an emerging need to develop PROMs for populations with cognitive impairments, particularly in the field of rehabilitation. Kramer and Schwartz (2017) addressed the issues of cognitive accessibility during PROM development and put forward a paradigm and recommendations for future PROM development in rehabilitation.

Finally, the number of items, and the time required to complete the questionnaire, should be acceptable in length and not exceed the person's cognitive and emotional limits (Waters et al. 2009).

Who should rate the child's health in paediatrics?
In child healthcare, parents and caregivers have traditionally been the spokesperson(s) for their children and the decision-makers for interventions on their child. Until recently researchers and clinicians have suggested that caregivers would have sufficient objectivity to reflect the child's own perceptions. The children themselves were considered to be too immature and unreliable to report on their own health. Nonetheless, over the last two decades, children have been invited to participate actively in the development of PROMs using robust qualitative and quantitative research methodologies. These efforts have confirmed that from the cognitive age of approximately 8 years,

children can independently, accurately, and reliably report about their own health, attitudes, and feelings (Ronen et al. 2003, Riley 2004). Today, PROMs are considered the criterion standard to evaluate persons with impairments and disability, even when they are children (Ronen 2016).

Researchers have identified repeatedly that children's self-reports and parents' proxy reports are not always concordant. A number of causes for discrepancy among raters have been explored. It appears that the reasons for this discrepancy stem from sub-jective personal realities, perceptions, valuation and views by the reporting person. One is the depression distortion hypothesis, whereby raters with depression (self or proxy) tend to score poorer on numerous health variables (Kendall et al. 1990, Richters & Pellegrini 1989, Eom et al. 2016). This observation is important because levels of anxiety and depression are likely to be higher among parents with a child/young person who has a chronic medical illness and higher still if their child/young person has emotional–behavioural problems (De los Reyes et al. 2011). In fact, Macleod and colleagues (1999) showed that the prevalence of mood disorders var-ied significantly by both informer and setting (i.e. clinical or community). Another potential cause is the concept of the disability paradox (Albrecht & Devlieger 1999) where some persons with impairments, apparently against all (externally perceived) odds, report that they are satisfied with their life and rate their health similar to typ-ical individuals, while external assessors are more negative (Ronen & Streiner 2013, 2016). The disability paradox is just one example of a more general phenomenon called response shift, in which people adapt to a change in state and this becomes their new normal (Streiner et al. 2015) – one with which (by their own judgment) they can apparently live well.

Returning to the scenario

Cassandra reviewed mounds of literature confirming the value of the ICF as an international classification system of functioning that allows health professionals to carefully map individuals' problems, needs, strengths, goal setting and guide interventions into the higher-level domains and dimensions of functions/impairments, activities/limitations, participation/restriction, and contextual facilitators/barriers. However, Cassandra also understood that the ICF is only the beginning of a new era in healthcare, wherein professionals should increasingly be required to demonstrate the impact of their services and intervention on people's functioning as reported by the people themselves. It became clear to Cassandra that applying children's PROMs would empower children to identify and address their own needs, thus incorporating the recommenda-tions by the United Nations Convention on the Rights of the Child (1989) and the Convention on the Rights of Persons with Disabilities (2006). She recognised that the earlier colleagues in her own and other institutions saw the importance of integrating the patients' perspectives into clinical practice, the easier would be the transition to a world where measuring the outcomes of services will become mandatory.

Cassandra also became aware that there are many challenges to overcome in trying to match the ICF with PROMs. Major steps, including knowledge translation, education and further health services research, will all be required to increase confidence in the added value of using PROMs to evaluate interventions from the patients' perspectives. Currently, PROMs are often routinely integrated into randomised clinical trials to assess whether treatment effects are evidence-based as far as patients are concerned, but are not routinely used in regular clinical care.

Cassandra decided to start, at her own institution, to work towards overcoming identified barriers for the clinical integration of PROMs and hoped that her efforts would be recognised and accepted. The barriers she identified included: (1) negative attitudes among clinicians towards collecting data or any evidence-based recommendations (she remembered that it took over 20 years for clinicians to follow the recommendations for parents to change babies' sleep position from prone to supine to reduce their risk for sudden infant death), or the ongoing opposition to vaccines by a large number of physicians; (2) the perception of the complexity of routine data collection, its integration and methodology; (3) tension among stakeholders when using or wishing to use PROM data for different purposes; and (4) concerns about confidentiality (Van der Wees et al. 2014).

Future opportunities

A cautionary note

Much can be done to introduce PROMs systematically into the daily clinical practice of health professionals. However, this should be done only once one can ensure that PROMs will achieve their goals. Research is still needed to evaluate the interventional effects of using PROMs over time (Antunes et al. 2014). In their critical book *Ending Medical Reversal*, Prasad and Cifu (2015) analysed how system interventions can go wrong. These authors have recognised that system interventions in healthcare are often adopted without a real plan to study them, and they note that once adopted, these systems become the 'standard of care' and can be very difficult to modify. In fact, some of these ineffective systems may even become mandated at a national level. Any system needs to show that it is actually effective, and does more good than harm, before being adopted. What is usually missing in healthcare is a system of continuous program evaluation and re-evaluation, with a willingness to abandon what does not work. So far, there is only weak evidence that, irrespective of the context of chronic conditions, PROMs have had at best a modest effect on developing or changing services, programs or interventions that have impacted patient outcomes (Boyce & Browne 2013, Kotronoulas et al. 2014).

The challenges of using PROMs in practice

Despite the presence of qualitative and quantitative studies examining various facilitators and barriers for a wider use of PROMs in our everyday practice, we still lack a set of universally accepted measures for a comprehensive measurement of PROs, addressing all aspects of health that are important to patients. Existing and future PROMs need better integration into clinical care, and must be tailored to the characteristics of each national healthcare system. Enabling the sustainable use of PROMs will require the shared vision of clinical professionals, purchasers, and patients, with a prudent selection of the steps to implement PROMs that will maximise their impact on the quality of healthcare. PROMs can be used as indicators to evaluate the effect of novel products and interventions, select treatments, evaluate quality of care, and monitor the health of individuals and populations. However, standards are needed regarding how PROMs are selected, collected, interpreted, reported and merged with other databases, to ensure that results are valid and meaningful for clinical care and policy decision-making (Black et al. 2016). In order to obtain high response rates from patients PROMs need to be quick and easy to administer and easy to score, and should provide useful clinical information (Duncan & Murray 2012). Practical recommendations require the dates of completion of questionnaires and the interventions of interest, as these are crucial to future longitudinal outcomes analysis. In addition, the data should be stored in a database that allows for immediate statistical analysis and with variables appropriately labelled to minimise additional complexities (Dawson et al. 2010).

Focus groups of parents (Tadic et al. 2012) identified the following aspects of parental experiences: (1) the importance of communication and the provision of information, more specifically information regarding the purpose of the questionnaire: What is it being used for and where is this information going? Also needed is a precise explanation: Why are the responses essential? Likewise, there is a need for feedback after completing a questionnaire to demonstrate that the responses and opinions are looked at and used, for example, to monitor progress. (2) User-friendly questionnaires are needed for gathering information: parents and children prefer short, clear and simple questionnaires but also more specific questionnaires that address their own issues in detail. As mentioned earlier, negative phrasing like 'Do you have trouble …' or phrasing that focuses exclusively on the person's difficulties may put people off giving candid responses. (3) Additional considerations include: fear of repercussion on the child's care and/or being judged as bad parents.

Importantly, using PROMs may encourage individuals to participate actively in their own healthcare. Today the PROMIS measurement system, still in its infancy, provides a set of common metrics to which PROMs that assess comparable constructs can be scaled.

Each PROMIS measure undergoes item response theory calibration and national norming of the calibrated scale to a mean of 50 and standard deviation of 10. Any item or scale that measures the same domain as a given PROMIS measure can be transformed to the PROMIS T-score, allowing users to collect data using the measure of their choice, but rendering it on a common metric (Black et al. 2016).

Towards successful implementations of PROMs
Clinicians have raised a number of concerns about introducing PROMs; these are summarised in systematic reviews, as well as qualitative and mixed studies. In their review on 'barriers and facilitators to routine outcome measurement by allied health professionals in practice' Duncan and Murray (2012) identified four high-level themes: (1) knowledge, education and perceived value in outcome measurement by professionals; (2) support/priority for the use of outcome measures; (3) practical considerations; and (4) patient considerations. It goes without saying that the educational component prior to the implementation is crucial. Duncan and Murray (2012) concluded that successful implementation of PROMs should be tailored by identifying and addressing the potential barriers (and facilitators) according to the specific setting and population. For example, having a coordinator throughout the implementation process seems to be key. The ongoing cognitive and emotional processes of each individual should be taken into consideration during changes. This could promote ownership and correct use of the measure by clinicians, potentially improving practice and the quality of care provided through use of PROMs data in clinical decision-making. Recently, papers have reported successful implementations of PROMs in practice using advanced technological systems (Jensen et al. 2015). Black and colleagues (2016) identified a number of gaps in PROMs applications and suggested introducing better strategies, including (1) guidance on how to select measures; (2) standardisation of metrics to facilitate comparisons; (3) interpretation of scores to help in clinical decisions; (4) identifying effective formats for feedback of the scored responses to patients and the healthcare systems that would follow with appropriate actions; and (5) developing an infrastructure for how to merge and access data from different sources.

Potential facilitators for the integration of PROMs into standard clinical service can be divided into three related programs, namely: preparation, implementation and evaluation (Antunes et al. 2014, Van der Wees et al. 2014):

- Preparation:
  - Develop a shared vision among patients, clinicians and policy makers.
  - Collect data to guide clinical care decisions.
  - Undertake knowledge translation and education about:
    - the prospect to enable clinicians to focus on patients' individual health goals and guide investigation and management decisions;

- the prospect for future comparative effectiveness studies;

- efforts towards clinical improvement at population or program levels.

- Implementation:

  - Implementation in countries with a single-payer health system would be easier than in countries with different private health sectors.

  - Involve a coordinator for the process.

  - Train people on how to use, interpret and present PROMs in clinical practice.

  - Develop an optimal order of steps needed for a successful implementation program.

  - Promote ownership of the measures at the level of management, health providers and patients.

  - Engage stakeholders to promote PROMs implementation and enable sustainability.

  - Integrate PROM data into electronic health records.

- Evaluation:

  - Provision of feedback from all stakeholders improves awareness of unmet needs and helps clinicians address specific patients' needs.

Conclusions

The ICF currently stands in the centre of international classification and terminology systems of health as viewed through the lens of functioning. The ICF can be expanded through its contextual factors to more explicitly include related dimensions such as QoL and spirituality that are important to patients and can be evaluated by patients themselves – they are, after all, the real experts on their own lives. People's self-reports of their own health, beyond the biological and physiological aspects that are the traditional focus of the healthcare system, are gaining recognition among policy makers and healthcare providers as criteria for measuring the effectiveness of programs, services and interventions, old and new. Clinicians will then be able to follow the different dimensions of health through routine periodic applications of PROMs. For ease of use PROMs can also be integrated electronically to allow this longitudinal surveillance of individuals and populations (see also Chapter 10). We may well be entering a new era of enhanced use of PROMs in clinical medicine, including rehabilitation, that will enable us to measure what is important to patients, using their assessments as our yardstick and providing guidance for our interventions and services. Future steps must include knowledge translation to make PROMs and their use easily understood, improve accessibility, practicality and feasibility of PROMs to fit the need of our patients, and promote their integration into daily clinical practice. Above all, research is needed to evaluate whether using PROMs makes a difference to patients, clinicians and the health systems in which they are engaged (Black et al. 2016). These are only a few of the opportunities for future research, education and development of program evaluations.

Acknowledgements

My sincere thanks to David Streiner PhD McMaster University, Hamilton, Ontario and the other editors of this volume for their constructive suggestions, recommendations and edits.

References

A De Los Reyes EA, Youngstrom SC, Pabo'n JK, Youngstrom NC, Feeny RL (2011) Findling Internal consistency and associated characteristics of informant discrepancies in clinic referred youths age 11 to 17 years. *J Clin Child Adolesc Psychol*, **40**: 36–53.

Albrecht GL, Devlieger PJ (1999) The disability paradox: highly qualified of life against all odds. *Soc Sci Med* **48**: 977–988.

Antunes B, Harding R, Higginson IJ (2014) Implementing patient-reported outcome measures in palliative care clinical practice: A systematic review of facilitators and barriers. *Palliat Med* **28**(2): 158–175.

Beauchamp T, Childress JF (eds.) (2013) *Principles of Biomedical Ethics, 7th edn*. New York: Oxford University Press.

Black N, Burke L, Forrest CB, et al. (2016) Patient-reported outcomes: pathways to better health better services and better societies. *Qual Life Res* **25**(5): 1103–1112.

Boyce MB, Browne JP (2013) Does providing feedback on patient-reported outcomes to healthcare professionals result in better outcomes for patients? A systematic review. *Qual Life Res* **22**(9): 2265–78.

Centers for Disease Control and Prevention (2015) CDC: 53 million adults in the US live with a disability [online]. https://www.cdc.gov/media/releases/2015/p0730-us-disability.html.

Chien CW, Rodger S, Copley J, Skorka K (2014) Comparative content review of children's participation measures using the International Classification of Functioning Disability and Health-Children and Youth. *Arch Physical Med Rehabil* **95**(1): 141–152.

Cieza A, Stucki G (2005) Content comparison of health-related quality of life (HRQoL) instruments based on the International Classification of Functioning disability and health (ICF). *Qual Life Res* **14**(5): 1225–1237.

Dawson J, Doll H, Fitzpatrick R, Jenkinson C, Carr AJ (2010) The routine use of patient reported outcome measures in healthcare settings. *BMJ* **340**: c186–c186.

Duncan EA, Murray J (2012) The barriers and facilitators to routine outcome measurement by allied health professionals in practice: a systematic review. *BMC Health Services Research* **12**: 96.

Eom S, Caplan R, Berg AT (2016) Behavioral Problems and Childhood Epilepsy: Parent vs Child Perspectives. *J Pediatr* **179**: 233–239.

eProvide (2002) Quality of Life Instruments Database – PROQOLID [online] https://eprovide. mapi-trust.org/about/about-proqolid.

Fayed N (2013) Practical considerations in choosing health health-related quality of life and quality of life measures for children and young people. In: Ronen GM, Rosenbaum PL (eds.) *Life Quality Outcomes in Children and Young People with Neurological and Developmental Conditions: Concepts Evidence and Practice.* London: Mac Keith Press, pp. 206–220.

Fayed N, Kraus de Camargo O, Kerr E, et al. (2012) Generic patient-reported outcomes in child health research: A review of conceptual content using World Health Organization definitions. *Dev Med Child Neurol* 54(12): 1085–1095.

Ferro MA, Avery L, Fayed N, et al. (2017) Child and parent-reported quality of life trajectories in children with epilepsy. *Epilepsia* 58: 1277–1286.

Geyh S, Schwegler U, Peter C, Müller R (2018) Representing and organizing information to describe the lived experience of health from a personal factors perspective in the light of the International Classification of Functioning Disability and Health (ICF): a discussion paper. *Disabil Rehabil* 6: 1–12

Grotkamp S, Cibis W, Behrens J, et al. (2010) Personbezogene Faktoren der ICF – Entwurf der AG 'ICF' des Fachbereichs II der Deutschen Gesellschaft für Sozialmedizin und Prävention [Personal contextual factors of the ICF draft from the Working Group 'ICF' of Specialty Group II of the German Society for Social Medicine and Prevention]. Gesundheitswesen 72(12): 908–916.

Grotkamp SL, Cibis WM, Nüchtern EAM, von Mittelstaedt G, Seger WKF (2012) Personal factors in the International Classification of Functioning Disability and Health: Prospective evidence. Australian J Rehabil Counsel 18(01): 1–24.

Grotkamp S, Cibis W, Bahemann A, et al. (2014) Bedeutung der personbezogenen Faktoren der ICF für die Nutzung in der praktischen Sozialmedizin und Rehabilitation [Relevance of Personal Contextual Factors of the ICF for Use in Practical Social Medicine and Rehabilitation]. Gesundheitswesen 76: 172–180.

Huber M, Knottnerus JA, Green L, et al. (2011) How should we define health? *BMJ* 343: d4163.

Huber M van Vliet M, Giezenberg M, et al. (2016) Towards a 'patient-centred' operationalisation of the new dynamic concept of health: a mixed methods study. *BMJ Open* 6(1): e010091.

Hutchings A, Neuburger J, Grosse Frie K, Black N, van der Meulen J (2012) Factors associated with non-response in routine use of patient reported outcome measures after elective surgery in England. *Health Qual Life Outcomes* 10(1): 34.

Janssens A, Thompson Coon J, Rogers M, et al. (2015) A systematic review of generic multidimensional patient-reported outcome measures for children part I: Descriptive characteristics. *Val Health* 18(2): 315–333.

Jensen RE, Rothrock NE, DeWitt EM, et al. (2015) The role of technical advances in the adoption and integration of patient-reported outcomes in clinical care. *Med Care* 53(2): 153–159.

Kendall PC, Stark KD, Adam T (1990) Cognitive deficit or cognitive distortion in childhood depression. *J Abnorm Child Phychol* 18(3): 255–270.

Kotronoulas G, Kearney N, Maguire R, et al. (2014) What is the value of the routine use of patient-reported outcome measures toward improvement of patient outcomes processes of care and health service outcomes in cancer care? A systematic review of controlled trials. *J Clin Oncol* 32(14): 1480–1501.

Kramer JM, Schwartz A (2017) Reducing barriers to patient-reported outcome measures for people with cognitive impairments. *Arch Physical Med Rehabil* 98(8): 1705–1715.

Kraus de Camargo O, Simon L 2013. *Die ICF-CY in der Praxis [Practical use of the ICF-CY]*. Bern: Verlag Hans Huber.

Mokkink LB, Terwee CB, Patrick DL, et al. (2010) The COSMIN study reached international consensus on taxonomy terminology and definitions of measurement properties for health-related patient-reported outcomes. *J Clin Epidemiol* **63**(7): 737–745.

MacLeod RJ, McNamee JE, Boyle MH, Offord DR, Friedrich M (1999) Identification of childhood psychiatric disorder by informant: comparisons of clinic and community samples. *Can J Psychiatry* **44**: 144–150.

Mayo NE. Dictionary of quality of life and health outcomes measurement. first edition. ISOQOL 2015.

Prasad VK, Cifu AS (2015) *Ending Medical Reversal: Improving Outcomes Saving Lives*. Baltimore: Johns Hopkins University Press.

Reynolds N, Mrug S, Wolfe K, Schwebel D, Wallander J (2016) Spiritual coping, psychosocial adjustment, and physical health in youth with chronic illness: a meta-analytic review. *Health Psychol Rev* **10**(2): 226–243.

Richters J, Pellegrini D (1989) Depressed mothers' judgments about their children : An examination of the depression – distortion hypothesis. *Child Dev* **60**(5): 1068–1075.

Riley AW (2004) Evidence that school-age children can self-report on their health. *Ambul Pediatr* **4**(4 Suppl): 371–376.

Riley WT, Rothrock N, Bruce B, et al. (2010) Patient-reported outcomes measurement information system (PROMIS) domain names and definitions revisions: further evaluation of content validity in IRT-derived item banks. *Qual Life Res* **19**(9): 1311–1321.

Ronen GM (2016) Patient-reported outcome measures in children with chronic health conditions: terminology and utility. *Dev Med Child Neurol* **58**(9): 896–897.

Ronen GM, Rosenbaum PL (eds.) (2013) *Health Participation and Quality of Life in Young People with Neurodevelopmental Conditions: Theory Concepts Evidence and Practice*. London: Wiley.

Ronen GM, Streiner DL (2013) Self-and proxy-rated valuations of outcomes. In: Ronen GM, Rosenbaum PL (eds.) *Life Quality Outcomes in Children and Young People with Neurological and Developmental Conditions: Concepts Evidence and Practice*. London: Mac Keith Press, pp. 234–248.

Ronen GM, Streiner DL (2016) Child- and parent-reported health: The Rashōmon effect of multiple realities. *J Pediatr* **179**: 17–18.

Ronen GM, Streiner DL, Rosenbaum P (2003) Health-related quality of life in children with epilepsy: development and validation of self-report and parent proxy measures. *Epilepsia* **44**(4): 598–612.

Sadeghi S, Fayed N, Ronen GM (2014) Patient-reported outcome measures in pediatric epilepsy: A content analysis using World Health Organization definitions. *Epilepsia* **55**(9): 1431–1437.

Schiariti V, Klassen AF, Cieza A, et al. (2014) Comparing contents of outcome measures in cerebral palsy using the International Classification of Functioning (ICF-CY): A systematic review. *Eur J Paed Neurol* **18**(1): 1–12.

Streiner DL, Norman GR, Cairney J (2015) *Health Measurement Scales: A Practical Guide to Their Development and Use*. Oxford: Oxford University Press.

Stucki G, Kostanjsek N, Ustün B, Cieza A (2008) ICF-based classification and measurement of functioning. *Eur J Phys Rehabil Med* **44**(3): 315–328.

Tadic V, Knowles RL, Rahi JS (2012) *Patient Reported Outcome and Experience Measures (PROMs and PREMs): Service Users' Perspectives.* London: Paediatric PROM&PREM Network.

United Nations (UN) (1948) *Constitution of the World Health Organization.* New York: United Nations.

Valderas JM, Alonso J (2008) Patient reported outcome measures: A model-based classification system for research and clinical practice. *Qual Life Res* **17**(9): 1125–1135.

Van der Wees PJ, Nijhuis-van der Sanden MWG, Ayanian JZ, et al. (2014) Integrating the use of patient-reported outcomes for both clinical practice and performance measurement: Views of experts from 3 countries. *Milbank Q* **92**(4): 754–775.

Wallander JL, Koot HM (2016) Quality of life in children: A critical examination of concepts, approaches, issues, and future directions. *Clin Psychol Rev* **45**: 131–143.

Waters E, Davis E, Ronen GM, Rosenbaum P, Livingston M, Saigal S (2009) Quality of life instruments for children and adolescents with neurodisabilities: how to choose the appropriate instrument. Dev Med Child Neurol 51(8): 660–669.

WHO (World Health Organization) (2007) *International Classification of Functioning Disability and Health – Children and Youth Version, 1st edn.* Geneva: World Health Organization.

WHO (World Health Organization) (1980) *International Classification of Impairments Disabilities and Handicaps (ICIDH) – A Manual of Classification Relating to the Consequences of Disease.* Geneva: World Health Organization.

Wilson IB, Cleary PD (1995) Linking clinical variables with health-related quality of life: a conceptual model of patient outcomes. *JAMA* **273**(1): 59–65.

Section B

Chapter 5

The ICF in clinical practice: Case scenarios and exercises

Liane Simon and Olaf Kraus de Camargo

Different degrees of detail and information can be conveyed using the ICF. This can be compared to the different levels at which music can be appreciated. One can enjoy listening to music, have a basic understanding of themes, melodies and rhythms; one can be able to read sheet music; and one might even be able to play an instrument or conduct an orchestra. For western classical music, all those activities rely on common conventions of how to annotate music and communicate it within a standard system. One cannot really appreciate the music simply by reciting the name of single notes or chords.

This also holds true for the ICF. For this reason, we encourage users of the ICF – and readers of ICF-based reports – to be aware that the use of the ICF codes alone is not enough. As we have tried to illustrate throughout this book, people's use of the ICF must be informed by an appropriate understanding and application of the concepts behind the language and the codes – and a clear idea of what purpose is being served by using the ICF. The ICF is by no means intended to be a secret code or jargon for specialists! The codes and definitions for each item, created by international consensus, serve as a reference and allow documentation of the functional profile of a person in context in a standardised way. This facilitates the exchange and analysis required to communicate about the populations we serve.

In addition, but different from western classical music, the use of the ICF is not meant to be linear. The framework illustrates this with the arrows between the components all being bidirectional. The way the framework has been published, readers tend to follow

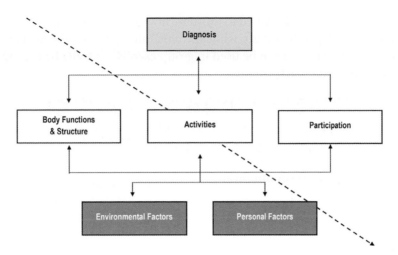

Figure 5.1 Conventional reading of the ICF.
Adapted from WHO 2007

it like they read a (western language) text – starting from the top left (see Fig. 5.1). This is a remnant from the predecessor of the ICF, the ICIDH, with the linear sequence 'disease → impairment → disability → handicap'. To be able to read the ICF from different directions it might be helpful to flip around the ICF framework, as illustrated below in Figure 5.2:

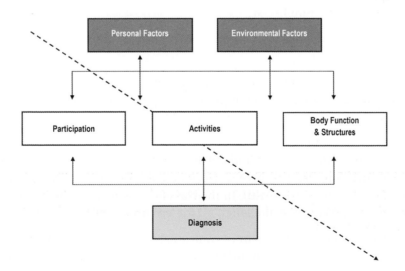

Figure 5.2 Person-centred approach to the ICF
Adapted from WHO 2007

Five learning objectives are described to illustrate how to work with the ICF. The first two are achievable by independent study, while the remaining three require the participation of other team members, and can be used in group exercises, ideally by colleagues with a variety of professional backgrounds.

- Objective 1: Knowledge of the five components of the ICF framework.

- Objective 2: Description of a functional profile based on the ICF.

- Objective 3: Interdisciplinary exchange based on the ICF.

- Objective 4: Courage to communicate.

- Objective 5: Goal formulation.

Objective 1: Knowledge and application of the five components of the ICF framework

The following are brief definitions of the components of the ICF:

- Body functions: the physiologic functions of body systems (including psychological functions). In the classification system, the items in this component are all preceded by the letter 'b' (for 'body').

- Body structures: the anatomical parts of the body such as organs, limbs and their parts. In the classification system, the items in this component are all preceded by the letter 's' (for 'structure').

- Activities: the execution of a task or action by a person. (These items are not classified separately, see below.)

- Participation: 'involvement in a life situation' while executing a task or action. In the classification system, the items for activities and participation are preceded by the letter 'd' for 'domain' as they are related to different life domains.

- Environmental factors: these are part of the contextual factors and comprise the elements of the material, social and behavioural surroundings. This element also includes domains to describe how services, systems and policies serve as barriers or facilitators to a person's health. In the classification system, the items in this component are preceded by the letter 'e' (for 'environment').

- Personal factors: these also are part of contextual factors. These elements describe the personal characteristics of an individual such as age, sex, education, religion, life style, motivation, ideas, fears, expectations, hope, sense of belonging or genetic predisposition. These items are not classified in the ICF.

Throughout this chapter the authors use an anonymised report of a boy we will call 'Dirk' to describe how we recommend the ICF framework, concepts and codes can be used. We first present a text report of the case, and then 'parse' the story using the elements of the ICF framework to illustrate where and how the several threads of the story can be grouped and then cross-linked. Following this exercise, we describe the thinking in which we engaged as we discussed both the aggregation of the 'pieces' and the kinds of questions that might arise as people do an exercise such as this one. While we do not offer any specific answer to Dirk's predicament, we hope that readers will see how the approach we are offering can be applied to any clinical situation and hopefully enrich clinical activities and interdisciplinary teamwork.

Dirk (male aged 4 years 11 months)

- *Read the report below and identify the elements that can be associated with the components of the ICF.*

- *Write those into the framework in two columns, one for* strengths/facilitators *and one for* difficulties/barriers.

Case analysis per ICF concepts
Dirk's parents were concerned about their son's development. The assessment information reported here was based on observations at the home of the family, in Dirk's kindergarten and by telephone with other professionals involved in the care of Dirk.

The discussion of goals involved the parents, his early intervention specialist, his paediatrician and his kindergarten teacher.

History
Dirk is his parents' only child and lives with them. He is turning 5 years old.

He was born preterm at 29 weeks of gestation by C-section. His weight was 1 285g, his length 41cm and his head circumference 27cm. The medical care occurred in the hospital, and a detailed discharge report was provided.

Dirk's paediatrician prescribed physiotherapy after discharge from the NICU due to a motor development problem. He was discharged from physiotherapy when he could walk independently at the age of 2 years.

In Germany, children are entitled to receive 10 preventive check-up examinations (identified by the letter U followed by a number) to detect chronic health conditions and developmental delays. The first one is done directly after birth, the last one at the age of five (U1 to U9, including U7a) (Institute for Quality and Efficiency in Health Care n.d.) During the last developmental check-up (U8), Dirk's paediatrician identified concerns with drawing and printing as well as attention problems.

Problem description

The parents report that they struggle a lot with Dirk's activity level. They describe him as loud and fidgety and report his ongoing fine motor difficulties with getting dressed and using cutlery. Dirk is not able to focus for a period on one task; his play is interrupted by constantly switching activities; and he requires a lot of attention from his parents. The parents report that they frequently feel overwhelmed and do not know how to support Dirk. Both seem very supportive and engaged and are trying to do their best to help their son.

During the mornings, Dirk attends kindergarten, while during the afternoons he is being cared for by his father, who has his own health and motor limitations. His mother works full-time and has not much time for Dirk. The family receives some support from Dirk's grandparents. A while ago they had trouble with their neighbours who complained of the boy's noise and called the local children's aid agency. An unannounced visit of an agency representative did not determine any risk of harm for Dirk.

According to his parents, Dirk has chronic hearing problems and has had repeated hearing tests. They report that since Dirk received ventilation tubes in his ears 9 months ago, he speaks in a lower volume and his speech development has improved.

Observation

Dirk is a friendly boy and quite confident in his interactions with his parents. During the visit to his home he is initially reserved but then seems to feel more assured and becomes more restless. He frequently provokes his parents with silly behaviours. His cognitive skills seem age appropriate. His posture seems hypotonic and he likes to rough-play. His father reports that he frequently takes him to a nearby playground and there he sometimes meets another boy and they play together.

To further assess his needs for early intervention, an observation in his kindergarten took place, and an interview with his teacher was done.

Dirk seems to enjoy being in the kindergarten group. He plays with younger children that seem to be more at his level of play skills. He talks very little. During play he prefers a broad base, lying on the floor or assuming a 4-point position. He seeks physical boundaries, crawls under tables and likes narrow spaces. His movements are not well coordinated. He does better when executing them quickly. He seeks proprioceptive stimuli and enjoys little play-fights with other boys, while always being friendly and attentive to the needs of others. His favourite activity is rough-play. He has good analytical and planning skills when building things.

He struggles with age-appropriate fine motor tasks and avoids those. His pencil grip is still palmar, he applies excessive pressure and struggles in calibrating his grip strength while manipulating play dough.

His teacher reports that he also struggles with chewing and swallowing. She has noticed some improvement, but he still eats only small bites and prefers soft foods.

He has no friends to play when outside of the kindergarten setting.

Steps 1 and 2
The first step is to become familiar with the components of the ICF. When reading the report, it can be helpful to use different coloured markers, one colour for each component, and go through the text identifying the related passages. Below you will find the relevant components we identified when going over this report. In undertaking this exercise in our clinic, we use a table that starts with Personal Factors and Environment, following the natural flow when describing a person in their environment. Then we describe Participation, followed by Activities and Body Functions/Structures (Table 5.1).

ISSUE: Parents of this only child (age 4y 9m) are feeling overwhelmed by their son's activity level and are wondering how to handle him.

Note that the section for Personal Factors does not make a distinction between Strengths and Challenges, as Personal Factors are not classified in the ICF as other components are. We strongly believe that it is important to annotate these, as they might help when proceeding with shared decision-making about goals for supports and interventions. Some topics might also be assigned to different components as depicted above. One might disagree on what constitutes a Personal Factor or a Body Function (e.g. is boisterous behaviour a lack of impulse control or a personal quality of being extroverted? Is the preference for narrow spaces just that, a preference, or a sensory-seeking behaviour?). It is sometimes difficult to tease apart the description of an Activity or Participation, in the sense of 'doing' as opposed to 'being involved' in a situation and executing such activity. These differences of interpretation (sometimes active disagreements) will require further discussion among the team members and the use of the ICF book (WHO 2001), ICF browser (http://apps.who.int/classifications/icfbrowser/) or available code sets (see Appendix 6) to verify the definitions and the inclusion and exclusion criteria for specific items.

Step 3 What else would you want to know and what suggestions do you have?
The answers to these questions depend on the hypotheses team members have generated to explain the issues described. These hypotheses usually are broader than diagnostic terms (in this case example, diagnoses such as 'Learning disability', 'Hearing loss', 'Attention-deficit–hyperactivity disorder',and 'Developmental coordination

Table 5.1 Overview of the findings organised by ICF topics

ICF Components	Strengths/Facilitators	Issues/Barriers
Personal Factors	<ul><li>Boy</li><li>Only child</li><li>Almost 5 years old</li><li>Born preterm at 29 weeks</li><li>Friendly and confident</li><li>Good cognitive skills</li><li>Initially reserved, but then more assured, becoming restless</li><li>Provokes parents with silly behaviours</li><li>Seems to like and seek narrow spaces and physical boundaries</li></ul>	
Environmental Factors, including human and physical supports	<ul><li>**Parents** very engaged and supportive, and want to help</li><li>Maternal grandparents are supportive</li><li>Attends half-day **kindergarten**</li><li>**Father** is afternoon caregiver</li><li>**Several professionals** are or have been involved</li><li>Paediatrician</li><li>Early intervention specialist</li><li>Kindergarten teacher</li><li>Social worker</li><li>Nearby playground</li><li>Ventilation tubes apparently improved hearing</li><li>Mother has full-time work</li><li>Children's services investigated and cleared Dirk and his family</li></ul>	<ul><li>Father has health problems</li><li>Mother work long hours</li><li>Neighbours have complained about Dirk's boisterous behaviour</li></ul>
Participation/ Activities	<ul><li>Good interaction with his parents</li><li>At the playground, plays well with another boy</li><li>Attends and enjoys kindergarten</li><li>Friendly and attentive to other children</li></ul>	<ul><li>No friends outside of kindergarten</li><li>Plays with younger children at kindergarten</li><li>Generally quiet at kindergarten – talking</li><li>'Silly behaviour'</li><li>Difficulties with:<ul><li>Dressing</li><li>Eating</li><li>Task completion</li><li>Printing</li><li>Chewing</li><li>Swallowing</li></ul></li></ul>

ICF Components	Strengths/Facilitators	Issues/Barriers
		• Delayed early motor development (walked at [or by] age 2 years) • 'Recent' concerns about drawing and writing skill challenges, as well as difficulties with activities of daily living (dressing, chewing and swallowing, using utensils) • Attention issues, loud and fidgety
Body structures/ functions	• Cognitive skills are age appropriate • Good analytic and planning skills	• Born preterm at 29/52, BWt = 1 285g (50th %ile), L = 41cm (90th %ile), HC = 27cm (50th %ile) • History of repeated hearing loss • Hypotonia and 'poorly coordinated movements'

disorder' might come to mind, all focused on specific body functions). However, given the remarkable heterogeneity of the manifestations of virtually all 'diagnoses', we are uncertain as to whether 'diagnosis' alone is helpful in identifying intervention goals. On the other hand, the view conveyed through the lens of the ICF allows for a 'diagnostic formulation' that includes the other ICF components as well. When elaborating a diagnostic formulation that will be helpful to develop goals and a plan to achieve them, additional information is often required. For the report above, such information could be:

• What is Dirk's neighbourhood like? Does it allow him to be outside? (Environmental Factor – physical)

• Are there other children to play with? (Environmental Factor – social)

• How do his grandparents feel about him? Are they also overwhelmed? (Environmental Factor – human)

• What have his parents/grandparents done so far to help him, and how is the relationship between them? (Environmental Factor – human)

- How much is the described lack of focus impacting his performance? Can he focus longer on tasks that require less fine motor skills or in a quiet environment? (Participation/Body Function/Environmental Factor)

- What is the availability of medication and community-based as well as clinical services? (Environmental Factors – services)

- School readiness? (Personal Factors – social and intellectual).

The diagnostic formulation could then be described as follows:

Dirk is a 5-year-old boy, single child of his parents, struggling with different activities like eating, dressing and printing that require fine motor coordination. He also struggles with verbal communication with his peers. He often presents with silly behaviours and does not stay on task for a long time, especially if it requires fine motor skills. His parents and grandparents are supportive and willing to help him. He enjoys the company of other children in the kindergarten class.

Suggestions for supports
As a first step, it would be helpful to explain to his teachers and family members the level of difficulty he has with fine motor skills (doing age-appropriate things with his hands) and the likelihood that these difficulties are frustrating to him. This will help them to understand the importance of coming up with supportive strategies that allow him greater participation and independence in those activities, perhaps doing things his own (alternative) way. Those strategies might be developed in cooperation with an occupational therapist. This approach might also sensitise his family to explore opportunities for social contact with other children that are not focused on competitive motor activities, but rather favour his strengths in visual–spatial thinking and analytic skills.

Objective 2: Description of a functional profile based on the ICF

For training purposes, we compiled anonymised clinical reports from clinician colleagues in this book. These reports have not necessarily been produced with the ICF in mind and the authors might have had different degrees of familiarity with the ICF. Most of the reports were produced by professionals working in German Early Intervention Centres or Social Paediatric Centres (Developmental Paediatric Services). Many were written with the goal of obtaining funding for Early Intervention for the patient described. In Germany, those funding decisions require a reference to the ICF.

As this book is intended for a broad audience, we are aware that the reports may not fulfil many of the various professional college standards for reporting patient information. At the end of this section we present a proposal for how an interprofessional and ICF-based report could look.

A frequent question asked during our workshops is: If the objective is a common language, why should we bother to find the right 'codes'? The answer we offer is that the codes are a short form for each of the concepts described in the items that compose the ICF. They make the ICF an international tool and anchor each item, even when translated into different languages. If everyone speaks the same language the codes should not be necessary. However, in our experience when discussing the description of the topics identified for a patient, even using the same language, it is not always clear and straightforward if people are talking about a structural lesion, an impaired function, or a limitation of activity/restriction of participation. Even environmental factors are not always clearly identified as such and a discussion can often develop about what constitutes a personal factor. In that discussion, it is helpful to consult the ICF description of the items as a reference and those items can be referred to consistently using the codes that identify each of the items. A familiarisation with the ICF definitions allows all members of the discussion to be 'on the same page'. This is an important step before starting the discussion about goals for intervention and support. Once clarity has been established about what constitutes a functional profile, people can debate which goals matter and are manageable with all the ICF dimensions involved. All these steps are easier to discuss by referring to the relevant codes describing the problem. The authors have provided, as an appendix to this chapter, some exercises that will enable people to try out the ideas described with the story of Dirk.

Objective 3: Interdisciplinary exchange based on the ICF

Identify colleagues that have worked with the same patient and ask them for a meeting. In our experience, we have organised such meetings in the following way:

One person presents the child and the family's story, ideally formulating a question to be answered at the end of the meeting. This discussion is structured as follows:

- clarify the team's questions;
- show a short video of the child (with consent of parents, clinicians record a home visit to share their impressions with the team);
- collect the resources of the family and the child;
- set identifiable goals;
- after agreement about the goals and precise description of the goals, code them with the corresponding ICF items for documentation purposes.

With such a procedure, the focus shifts to content and goals, and only at the end is the ICF used for coding purposes. Initially, the time requirements for preparation and meetings will probably be above the usual times available for you. After becoming comfortable with the ICF and having gone through several case discussions with your colleagues these time requirements will reduce. Until you reach that comfort level, try not to implement the ICF as a rule but only use it for single cases discussed during times available for Quality Improvement or team development, as a way of learning and teaching.

For a broader discussion about interprofessional practice and the ICF, see Chapter 6.

Once you have completed the first three objectives, we suggest two more be considered.

Objective 4: Courage to communicate

Not all professionals will have the time or interest to use the ICF to engage in an exchange about patients, especially if they are working outside our work place and are unfamiliar with these concepts. Therefore, you will need to be assertive and take the initiative to be a 'knowledge broker'. You will have a double duty: teaching ICF concepts, and having a case conference about a common patient. Having obtained consent from the parents, it is helpful to reach out to all the professionals involved with your patient, including people outside of your institution. Ask them what goals they would propose be achieved for the child and family in the next 6 months, whose goal it is, and why each goal is important, and add this information into the planning process. When communicating about goals, ask how these goals will improve participation and if there are any barriers to be considered. You do not need to lecture about the ICF, Domains, Chapters or Items. Making the discussion practical and oriented to the specific situation of the patient and the family allows people to relate to what you are trying to achieve. Once you have collected that information you can add it into the planning process, adding it for example in a filled-out framework with the items marked from your perspective and ask them to comment or add items they feel are missing. Below is another case study which provides an example of how such a situation could look.

Jonas 6y 8m, male

Jonas is 6 years and 8 months old when his parents bring him to our centre for a second opinion. He is an only child and lives with his parents in a single home.

Reason for the referral
In May of this year Jonas received a diagnosis of myoclonic dystonia (ICD 10: G24.1). His mother reports a genetic predisposition in her family. The parents brought several reports of consultations from other services and wanted a second opinion how to best support their son. He already receives occupational therapy twice and speech and language therapy once per week.

The parents report that they notice major difficulties executing fine motor skills in all activities of daily living. One major area of difficulty is getting dressed. All academic tasks dependent on those skills (printing, drawing, holding a pencil) are also a significant challenge for Jonas. During other activities such as playing with Lego or role play he does not have difficulties and shows great creativity and perseverance. On the other hand, they notice an increasing tendency to avoid activities that require more motor skills. Jonas continues with his friendly demeanour but ends up withdrawing himself from such situations.

The parents hope to obtain more ideas and information on how to deal with these difficulties. The amount and range of therapy already being done, and the concerns about the academic future of their son, occupy a significant amount of their family life. Jonas's parents assure us that they are willing to do anything needed to help their son but also want him to have enough free time to be able to do things on his own.

Observation
Jonas is a very friendly boy who has no difficulty in engaging in social contact with the examiners. He presents with low postural tone and speaks unclearly and with a nasal voice. The muscle strength in the upper and lower extremities is slightly reduced. Despite the articulatory difficulties, his language is understandable, and he impresses by using a large vocabulary for his age and building complex sentence structures. His cognitive skills seem age appropriate. During the assessment, he executes a series of fine motor activities and presents with a low-amplitude intention tremor. When asked to draw a picture he does not comply and instead redirects the examiner to another activity. His gross motor skills are clumsy and frequently accompanied by associated movements and co-contractions of the contra-lateral limbs. He can pass a cord only through a large opening of a big bead. When putting on his socks he grabs them with a palmar grip and takes a bit longer than expected to manage this task. His mother comments that at home they usually decide beforehand, depending on the availability of time, if he is going to dress himself or if she will dress him.

After you have collected the information above from the parents and have observed and examined Jonas, you decide to write up the main findings and issues according to the ICF in the form of a table as seen above, for the example 'Dirk' or you can also use the ICF framework as shown below (Fig. 5.3). You present this to the parents for further discussion.

This example illustrates that sometimes access to therapies does not necessarily mean that they will promote participation. Here the parents have requested a second opinion, and in the circumstances the treating therapists could not be involved in the discussion. As reported by the parents, the therapies did not seem to focus on real-life situations (in ICF terms the therapies were addressing issues at the level of body structure and function), and had required a significant amount of time from the family and the child over the last 2 years. Recognising Jonas' strengths and the

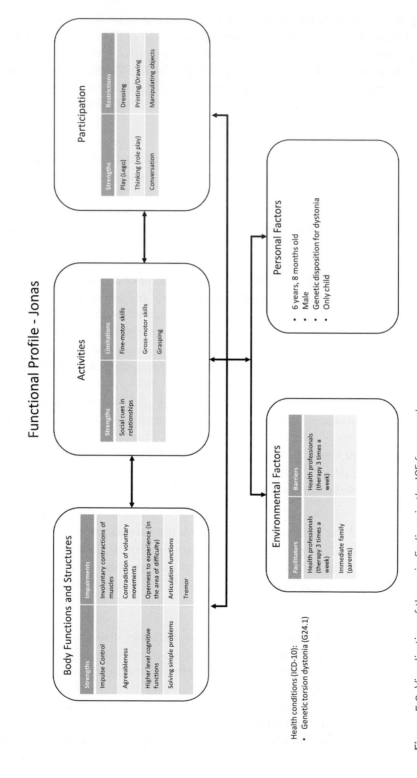

Figure 5.3 Visualisation of the main findings in the ICF framework
Adapted from WHO 2007

practical needs for him to be successful at school will be fundamental in supporting him. The energy of intervention should therefore be directed towards building on existing strengths and promoting the development of supportive relationships with peers and teachers while also facilitating the achievement of daily tasks in ways that are adaptive for Jonas, even if done differently.

Specific points of entry along the ICF and recommendations could be discussed with the other professionals involved. Being clear about the goals can help to have a non-judgmental discussion about the ways to achieve them most effectively for the child and the family. That way, the discussion becomes about Jonas and not about who is treating him. Below we have listed some goals for Jonas and his family and linked them to specific ICF categories:

Problem solving (D175)
Based on his coordinative difficulties Jonas will need to learn to develop coping and compensatory strategies. The occupational therapy should focus on those in collaboration with his parents and teachers to allow him to succeed academically according to his cognitive potential.

Products and technologies for education (e130)
At school, it will become more and more difficult for Jonas to produce legible texts in the amount of time available. He should have access to electronic text processing (PC, tablet, software) to help with this. The training of handwriting should be done independent of other academic tasks, and academic performance should not be judged by handwriting!

Support by health professionals (e355)
By focusing interventions on relevant activities for participation in school and at home, there should be a discussion with the treating therapists as to whether the frequency of current therapies could be reduced, with the newly 'freed' time being used by Jonas to meet and play with friends.

Public education (D817)
Jonas' teachers should be informed about his challenges and his needs for supports before he starts Grade 1. This would allow them to connect in time with the learning resource teacher to coordinate the strategies mentioned above.

Involuntary movements/muscle strength (b765)
The aetiology of the reported diagnosis and the relation to the clinical findings is not clear yet. Jonas parents have already booked an appointment at the dystonia clinic at the University and we are supportive of this. His coordination difficulties are very much in line with the difficulties experienced by children with Developmental

Coordination Disorder, but for that diagnosis other neurologic conditions need to be ruled out.

Objective 5: Goal formulation with the family and the team

Within the team, try to agree on a total but limited number of goals. It is important that all disciplines are aware of all the goals, and in our experience, it is also important to limit the number of goals (six goals are the absolute maximum). That way the goals can be kept in mind by everyone involved. On the other hand, it is important to be aware of all potential goals before reducing them to a manageable number for current intervention. This allows people to revisit them in future meetings and re-prioritise them. To prioritise, everyone involved (including the family, and the child where possible) needs to ask: 'What is the goal we want to reach first, for what reasons, and what is of greatest importance for the child and the family?' A guiding principle to answer these questions should be the aspect of goals enabling participation of the child and the family.

Many parents of children with neurodevelopmental disabilities state as their early goals that the child should learn to walk and talk. This is a very understandable desire, but professionals sometimes need to consider that such goals are still very far away or perhaps not ever attainable. It can be helpful to register the goal as expressed by the parents but then to introduce intermediate goals that are achievable and contribute to the parents' goal. (As an example, a communication system can enable a non-speaking child to express what they are thinking and wanting; thus, while 'talking' may not be happening yet, the functions attained by talking (i.e. 'communicating') can be!). One way to frame these ideas are the F-words tools developed at CanChild; for example, using the F-words goal sheet (Appendix 3).

The reports are descriptive, and the goals identified are the result of the opinions and discussions of other professionals and the family. They are intended as a basis for further discussion. The ICF framework provides an excellent means to describe a child and family's situation broadly in a biopsychosocial 'picture', but it is not an assessment tool and cannot substitute tools currently used by professionals to capture the details and nuances of a person's predicaments.

In this sense, the ICF as a common language can be considered a conceptual and communication tool. The process of generating reports should be collaborative to ensure that the formulated goals represent the opinion of the whole team involved. A different team might have a different set of goals; indeed, each reader might challenge which goals, in their opinion, should have been chosen for the example in the report. These opinions need to be discussed with the other team members that know the child and family to reach a consensus. The reports might not contain all the relevant information used for the discussion. Our intention is to demonstrate how – across disciplines – the ICF can be used. The examples should show that the interdisciplinary coordination does more than inform each other about the goals one might identify from the point of view of one's discipline. We recommend settling for a manageable number of goals commonly agreed upon with the family (and child where appropriate), that support them to become active and valued participants in the decision-making process. Appendix 7 contains a collection of tools and links.

References

Institut für Qualität und Wirtschaftlichkeit im Gesundheitswesen (IQWiG) [Institute for Quality and Efficiency in Healthcare] (n.d.). Welche Früherkennungsuntersuchungen werden von den gesetzlichen Krankenkassen bezahlt? [Which preventive exams are funded by public insurance?]. https://www.gesundheitsinformation.de/welche-frueherkennungsuntersuchungen-werden-von.2272.de.html. (Accessed on November 3rd, 2018)

WHO (World Health Organization) (2007). *International Classification of Functioning, Disability and Health – Children and Youth Version* (First). Geneva, Switzerland: WHO press. Retrieved from http://apps.who.int/iris/bitstream/10665/43737/1/9789241547321_eng.pdf.

Chapter 6

The development of effective health and social care teams: ICF as the glue!

Stefanus Snyman, Liane Simon and
Olaf Kraus de Camargo

The ICF is described as a multipurpose classification with four aims: (1) to provide a scientific basis for understanding and studying health; (2) to establish a common language to describe health; (3) to allow comparison of data across countries; and (4) to provide a systematic coding scheme for health information systems (WHO 2007). The aim of establishing a common language is fundamental for the development of interprofessional collaboration. 'Speaking ICF' should make it easier to talk with and understand each other. However, developing and speaking a new language is always influenced by cultural contexts. This applies equally to various professions and our often-separate professional languages. For this reason, using the ICF could help all of us to develop an interprofessional culture of goal setting.

In this chapter, we discuss (1) how goals can be understood from varied perspectives; (2) the need for interdisciplinary collaboration in establishing goals; (3) the impact of collaborative goal setting on team development; and (4) health professionals as 'environmental factors'. We take a closer look at these four themes, and explore the challenges and possibilities of each. We also comment on 'Hidden goals' and how these can be detected and considered.

The meaning of 'goals' and the different perspectives on problems

When people seek the help of a health professional they expect to get assistance to achieve a goal. The person themself, or somebody who cares for them (e.g. their parent), searches for the right professionals to help them. If there is a choice, patients want health professionals whom they perceive to be the best fit for their problem or for achieving their goals.

In the same light, every professional also tries to achieve goals, meaning that we too are trying to be goal-oriented. The question arises, however, as to whether patients and families, and health professionals, have the same goals; and even when they appear to agree on the goal, do they mean the same thing by those goals?

Searching for goals, but first defining the 'problem'
In many situations, goals are not clearly defined. They might vary from broadly stated goals (e.g. 'I am trying to find out what is going on') to very specific goals (e.g. 'I want a selective dorsal rhizotomy for my child'). Patients/clients and their stakeholders – hoping for advice from the professional – can easily be upset or frustrated when people ask them about their goals. In the spirit of the philosophy of family-centred service (FCS), one might argue that professionals *should* be engaging families in goal setting and decision-making about their issues in the context of the family's values and experiences. On the other hand, many families, especially early in their journey into the field of childhood disability, may be both overwhelmed by the challenges they face and as yet uncertain what goals might even be appropriate. From the perspective of FCS, it can be argued that supporting families who make the conscious decision to share, or even hand over, decision-making and goalsetting responsibility to professionals is entirely consistent with an FCS approach to service delivery, as long as it is indeed the family's decision.

But what kind of help has a positive impact? This, like the description of the problem itself, might be seen from different perspectives. Although everybody may think that they are talking about the same problem, this is often not the case. For this reason, searching for goals needs to be clearly based on the 'problem' that is being identified. We like to frame this as 'WTQ' (What's the Question?).

Sharing information to identify the problem
From a systemic point of view, clear articulation of problems is an important starting point towards potential solutions. If someone can clearly define something as a problem, they know that this issue is something that potentially could be different, and hopefully better. They usually will have an idea what 'better' could look like. However, when it comes to coping with, for example, one's diagnoses or health condition, one

first needs to get information not only from health professionals but from as many other sources as possible, in order to understand others' perspectives about possible resolutions of the dilemmas. This means that the first thing health professionals should do in a situation like this is to help the person to know enough about their overall situation, including 'possibilities'. This foundation of information forms a platform for the next step, which involves talking about the problem(s) and what kind of goals the person would like to pursue.

It is not always easy to talk about problems and ask for help towards the development of goals. It may be necessary to help patients to make their implicit goals explicit. Based on the obvious reality that we all see things through our own lenses, the self-identified problems might be different from the issues others have identified as the problem. Hence, common goal setting needs common problem identification and a well-captured mandate clarification between the person and the professional. Readers are referred to Chapter 5, in which we have presented several 'cases' with an ICF-based account and analysis.

Interdisciplinary collaboration

We should reinforce here that different issues need to be recognised as important in trying to bring ICF concepts to life with a vivid language. Healthcare professionals working with and for a person ('patient') become members of the team around the person. This team is often large and encompasses more persons than simply the team within an institution such as a clinic or a school. Therefore, interprofessional collaboration is needed, and this often requires interdisciplinary collaboration across sectors as well. And to make this issue even more challenging, inter-institutionality requires the collaboration of professionals working in/for different institutions that often have varied mandates. It is here that the ICF can provide the umbrella of a common framework and language under which everyone can gather.

Working together as a team depends on complementary competencies of team members (Hackmann 1990). Teams need to clarify their purpose and goals, their responsibilities and procedures. To be a member of a team around the 'patient' is something that needs to be carefully considered. To behave within this team in a facilitating way with persons not usually viewed as team members (e.g. parents, patients, teachers, pastors, community workers) presents both an amazing opportunity and a novel challenge for many people. This means, among other considerations, being aware of all professionals (and friends and family) who are important to and are working with the person and their family.

The idea of considering all of these players as members of the patient's team is a very challenging part of the philosophy of the biopsychosocial model. This is particularly true because some professions are acculturated to be the leader within a team, while others are conditioned to play a minor role. Furthermore, some professions have not traditionally learned to work together as a team. In light of these considerations, it is helpful to look at the principles underlying team development, with its different stages and forms of teams described in the literature:

Various terms are used to describe health and social care teams. Given the ongoing terminological uncertainty within the interprofessional field, great effort has gone into a global process to clarify various terms. Over the past decade these terms have evolved and a common understanding has been reached through work done by the Centre for the Advancement of Interprofessional Education (CAIPE) and the Journal of Interprofessional Care (2017) (Box 6.1).

Other organisations have approached this topic in similar ways. The Canadian Interprofessional Health Collaborative developed a competency framework to guide interprofessional education and collaborative practice for all professions in a variety of contexts (Canadian Interprofessional Health Collaborative 2010). This National Interprofessional Competency Framework provides an integrative approach to describe the competencies required for effective interprofessional collaboration. Six competency domains highlight the knowledge, skills, attitudes and values that shape the judgments essential for interprofessional collaborative practice. The six competency domains are:

1) interprofessional communication

2) patient/client/family /community-centred care

3) role clarification

4) team functioning

5) collaborative leadership

6) interprofessional conflict resolution.

Figure 6.1 illustrates how the last 4 domains contribute to interprofessional communication and the delivery of FCS.

Interprofessional communication

   Competency statement: Practitioners from different professions should communicate with each other in a collaborative, responsive and responsible manner.

On a meso level the ICF can be seen to represent the social structures providing connections between micro systems; for example, environmental factors such as connections

Box 6.1   Clarifying terminological uncertainty within the interprofessional field

Prefixes:

✓ *inter-* refers to working in a synchronised way, i.e. in terms of interdisciplinary – the occupational therapist, paediatrician and teacher are working together from the same hymn sheet.

✓ *multi-* refers to functioning in parallel, i.e. in terms of a multiprofessional approach to patient care, the doctor may refer to the physiotherapist, but they don't have an integrated management plan; they work in parallel.

Suffixes:

✓ *-disciplinary* refers to various academic disciplines such as health sciences, psychology, education, anthropology, economics, geography, political science, computer science, etc.

✓ *-professional* refers to health and social care professions such as nursing, medicine, pharmacy, physiotherapy, social work, etc.

Collaborative patient-centred practice is a type of arrangement designed to promote the participation of patients and their families within a context of care.

Collaboration is an active and ongoing partnership, often between people from diverse backgrounds, who work together to solve problems or provide services.

Interdisciplinary teamwork relates to the collaborative efforts undertaken by individuals from different disciplines such as health sciences, social work, psychology, anthropology, education, computer science, etc.

Interprofessional collaboration is a type of interprofessional work which involves different health and social care professions who regularly come together to solve problems or provide services, such as nursing, medicine, pharmacy, physiotherapy, social work, etc.

Interprofessional coordination is a type of work, similar to interprofessional collaboration (see above) as it involves different health and social care professions. It differs as it is a 'looser' form of working arrangement whereby interprofessional communication and discussion may be less frequent in nature.

Interprofessional teamwork is a type of work which involves different health and/or social professions who share a team identity and work closely together in an integrated and interdependent manner to solve problems and deliver services.

Intraprofessional is a term which describes any activity which is undertaken by individuals within the same profession, such as a paediatrician, surgeon and a family physician.

Multidisciplinary teamwork is an approach where the team members are composed from different academic disciplines (e.g. occupational therapy, psychology, sociology, mathematics) referring to each other and working in parallel without one integrated master plan.

Professions are occupational groups who in general provide services to others, such as nurses or social workers. The expression can be used as a term of self-ascription to avoid the need to apply regulatory criteria which differ between groups.

Transdisciplinary is an activity designed to promote generic working: a process whereby the activities of one discipline are undertaken by members of another, e.g. the teacher helps with the fine motor coordination traditionally done by the occupational therapist.

Transprofessional is an activity designed to promote generic working: a process whereby the activities of one professional group are undertaken by members of another, e.g. the nurse doing stump cone bandaging and not the physiotherapist.

Unidisciplinary is an activity undertaken by one discipline alone, e.g. education, medicine.

Terminology used by the Journal of Interprofessional Care 2017, reprinted with permission from Scott Reeves, editor-in-chief.

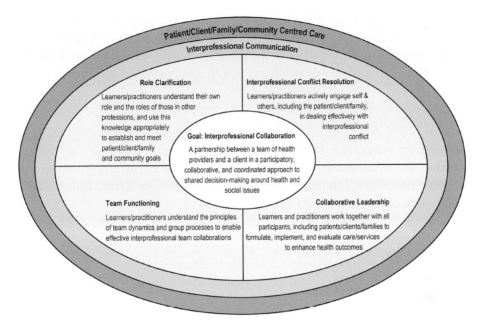

Figure 6.1 Canadian Interprofessional Health Collaborative's National Interprofessional Competency Framework
Adapted and reproduced with thanks to the Canadian Interprofessional Health Collaborative.

between a person's family and the neighbourhood, and between different members of the interprofessional team interacting with the service user. The service user is not participating directly in such processes, but is affected by them through direct contact with both other levels of these systems (Bronfenbrenner & Ceci 1994, Hollenweger 2010). On the meso level interprofessional collaborative practice competencies can be developed as the ICF is used as a conceptual framework and common language to interpret the narrative through interprofessional communication, person-centred teamwork, as well as ethical and value considerations.

Children with developmental disabilities frequently present with impairments of various organ systems and restrictions of participation in different life domains. They also come from various socio-economic backgrounds and are impacted by different attitudes, systems, services and policies. They are frequently connected to a variety of professionals within the disciplines of health and social care, but also within education. Interdisciplinary teams are also often part of the care of those children and their families. Those teams rely on reports from different disciplines for their team meetings and case discussions. In this context, the structure and nomenclature of the ICF can be useful to facilitate the understanding and communication among the professionals involved, by providing a transdisciplinary 'common' language to all. The ICF also makes it possible to include patients and caregivers more effectively in this process, resulting in recommendations that are based on shared, informed decision-making. Such a procedure results in reports using the language of the ICF, thus contributing to the implementation of the interventions and coordination of the different professionals involved in them.

Patient/client/family/community-centred care

> **Competency statement:** 'Learners/practitioners seek out, integrate and value, as a partner, the input and the engagement of the patient/client/family/community in designing and implementing care/services.' (https://www.cihc.ca/files/CIHC_IPCompetencies_Feb1210.pdf)

ICF serves as a catalyst for interdisciplinary person-centred collaboration on micro-, meso- and macro levels of systems for health. In describing these levels, it is assumed that the paradigm of the service is user-centred, and not provider- or profession-centred (Snyman et al. 2016).

The micro level can be described as the direct, lived experience of the service user, as they interact with student professionals, service providers, family, culture, worldviews and the system. This interaction is reciprocal – an iterative juggling progressing in complexity (Bronfenbrenner & Ceci 1994, Hugo & Couper 2006). ICF provides the common language and biopsychosocial approach for the interprofessional team to engage, clarify and interpret these narratives. In their discussions with children with disabilities and their parents, Rosenbaum and Gorter (2012) use 'F-words' (function, family, fun, friends, fitness and future) to explain and clarify the narrative in terms of the ICF components. We believe that the F-words illustrate one way to operationalise the ICF ideas.

Using ICF uniprofessionally or multiprofessionally challenges service providers and students to avoid viewing a service user in a narrow perspective as someone whose problems relate only to their individual profession or specific discipline. Rather, one is ethically committed to view the person within a biopsychosocial-spiritual context, realising that interdisciplinary collaboration, prioritisation, person-centred goal setting and outcomes reported by service users may all be needed to address needs. Taking cognisance of the person's activity limitations and participation restrictions, as well as the barriers and facilitators of environmental factors in light of personal factors, service providers and students gain a broader understanding of the person's health in context, and this emphasises the team's responsibility to move beyond siloed professional paradigms. This also highlights the need for a diverse team of healthcare professionals and represents a mind shift in how to approach health and healthcare (Winiarski 1997, Dufour & Lucy 2010, Snyman et al. 2015).

Role clarification

> **Competency statement:** Practitioners should understand their own role and the roles of those in other professions, and use this knowledge appropriately to establish and achieve patient/client/ family and community goals.

The ICF supports the exchanges among different disciplines and contributes to their cooperation. Such an exchange requires that the representatives of the different professions clarify their roles in the team and reach a mutual understanding of the theoretical backgrounds of the different professions. Not only can the theoretical backgrounds be different from one profession to another, but even within the same profession, depending on the era of training. Without going deeper into the theories of childhood development it is important to recognise that different professionals might have different backgrounds, attitudes and approaches that are grounded in theories from each of those disciplines. In order to collaborate productively it is important to acquire knowledge about each other's backgrounds. Some questions might arise:

- On which theoretical basis are we evaluating child development?

- What do we mean by 'developmental disability', 'developmental delay', 'developmental disorder' and 'normal development'?

- On the basis of which theory are we expecting a causal relationship between therapeutic or intervention efforts and child development?

- For which areas of the child's development are we responsible?

These questions are related to the background and relationship of each practitioner to their discipline, be it in the health or social sciences. This background also determines the understanding of evidence. Usually, we expect that our scientific understanding is the same across all disciplines and that knowledge and evidence generated have absolute value. When we say we 'know', we are basing our understanding on some 'truth' found in science that informs our professional training. But scientific 'truths' are generated by methods and rules that might differ between health and social sciences.

It is desirable, therefore, that we abandon a rigid separation of tasks and roles in the interest of collaboratively attending to the developmental needs of the child and the family. This can be achieved through regular communication among the different disciplines involved in care, to ensure everyone is on the same page for the best possible support for the child (Thurmair & Naggl 2000, Sohns 2000).

When utilising ICF, one realises that to enact a person-centred, integrated biopsychosocial approach involves actions that usually requires the expertise of more than one

Acute Care

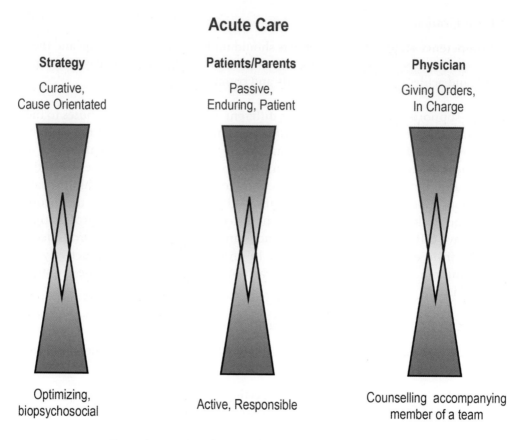

Strategy	Patients/Parents	Physician
Curative, Cause Orientated	Passive, Enduring, Patient	Giving Orders, In Charge
Optimizing, biopsychosocial	Active, Responsible	Counselling accompanying member of a team

Developmental Care/Early Intervention

Figure 6.2   Cultures of care, strategies, patient's and physician's roles

profession or discipline. It is therefore important to clarify roles as part of the process of becoming a high-performance team. It is important not only to clarify roles from a professional perspective, but also to recognise that roles often need to change due to the context in which the professional is working. For example, acute and developmental care differ with regards to the underlying 'culture', characterised by the approach or strategy that clinicians pursue with their interventions and the roles expected to be fulfilled by patients and physicians within each of those cultures (Figure 6.2).

Team functioning

Competency statement: Practitioners need to understand the principles of team-work dynamics and group/team processes to enable effective interdisciplinary collaboration.

The ICF requires the cooperation of different knowledgeable people, with their scientific backgrounds and methods, in order to use their knowledge collaboratively. Depending on the diversity of backgrounds, this cooperation is not always easy or natural. The opinions of individuals might not be shared by others and no scientific paradigm should hold sway over another. Interdisciplinary teamwork is required in order to overcome these challenges.

According to Sohns (2000):

> no specialist alone unifies all the necessary professional and human competencies required to support all children and all parents. Therefore, early intervention requires an interdisciplinary cooperation of specialists in order to benefit both, children and parents. In this sense, early intervention can be understood as an opportunity for the different specialists to develop trust into each other and assume a shared responsibility complementing each other's skills with their specific competencies.

The cooperation between specialists from the varied fields of pedagogy, medicine, psychology and therapy has the objective to facilitate an early establishment of supports that are holistic, manageable for the parents, as well as tailored to the needs of the child and family.

Collaborative leadership

Competency statement: Practitioners should understand and can apply leadership principles that support a collaborative practice model.

Once a decision is made to implement the ICF into a service model, there is usually an expectation that the quality of services will improve with improved interdisciplinary work. Such a quality improvement is not automatic, as it needs to address several barriers in order to be implemented. First, time for meetings and case discussions is usually limited, as the funding for developmental services is often linked to direct services to the clients, and so-called indirect services result in lower rates of reimbursement. In addition, there is a learning curve to be able to work collaboratively and bridge the disciplinary boundaries.

Collaborative leadership implies continued individual accountability for one's actions, responsibilities and roles as explicitly defined within one's professional/disciplinary scope of practice. To support interprofessional collaborative practice learners and practitioners collaboratively determine who will provide group leadership in any given situation by supporting the following:

• working with others to enable effective patient/client outcomes;

• advancement of interdependent working relationships among all participants;

- facilitation of effective team processes;

- facilitation of effective decision-making;

- establishment of a climate for collaborative practice among all participants;

- co-creation of a climate for shared leadership and collaborative practice;

- application of collaborative decision-making principles;

- integration of the principles of continuous quality improvement to work processes and outcomes (Canadian Interprofessional Health Collaborative 2010).

The ICF facilitates the knowledge contribution from different disciplines free from a hierarchical order. Team members working with the ICF must be empowered to feel free to express their opinions and observations regardless of their profession.

Interprofessional conflict resolution

Competency statement: Practitioners actively engage self and others, including the client/patient/family, in positively and constructively addressing disagreements as they arise.

One of the most frequent discussion points brought up during workshops on inter-professional collaboration are issues such as: 'Am I allowed to comment on language abilities, despite being a physiotherapist?' While this is an issue of role clarification, it is also deeply embedded in an underlying conflict, which can be positive, but can also be a negative. If such conflicts arise they put profession-centred self protectionism and possibly jealousy above patient-centredness. In going deeper into such discussions, many participants reveal that within their teams there exist quite strict rules as to who can address which areas of the development or skill of a child. We suspect that a significant part can be explained by insecurity about the own professional role; how it is valued within the team; and possibly previous negative experiences of cooperation. 'How far do I go as a professional?', 'What are my professional values and approaches?', 'How do they conflict with those of other professions?', 'What differentiates my profession from the others?', 'Am I willing to change my practice and convictions in the light of new information brought by other disciplines?'

Preconceived notions and anecdotal evidence about other professionals often prevail at the beginning of a phase of team development, and only after building open and trusting relationships those can be overcome. The ICF provides a common language that can facilitate this process by being used across the disciplines, expanding the own jargon. In this sense, the implementation of the ICF can be seen as catalyst for an inter- and transdisciplinary development of teams and reflective conflict resolution, which in turn can lead to trust-based task sharing and task shifting. As teams change over time, such processes of team development need to occur repeatedly when new members join.

On the *macro* level the ICF can also help to bridge the conflict that exists between the service providers on the ground and those responsible for policy development and service administration, as the ICF provides a mechanism for person-centred amalgamated data for the improvement of systems for health:

> There is hardly a more sensitive impact on the working climate than the one caused by disregard by colleagues. On the other hand, the most important condition for interdisciplinary understanding and cooperation is being competent in one's own area of practice (Speck 1996, p. 48, translation by the authors).

Team development

Teams are characterised by both external and internal factors. External factors can be a shared location, shared working times or meeting times; internal factors are defined by the team members, their personalities and their professional background, knowledge and skill set. To establish an interdisciplinary team, it is not enough to hire professionals from different disciplines and declare that they are going to work as a team. Teams develop over time by establishing a culture of rules of communication and responsibilities. This process of growth and dynamics has been divided into different phases. While these are theoretical constructs, understanding them might be helpful in analysing team processes, and supporting teams in their further development. The stages described below, and illustrated in Figure 6.3, are not necessarily sequential, and teams might become stuck in certain stages for different periods of time. Teams also are subject to changes with new members joining and long-time members leaving them. Such changes can initiate new phases of team development (Robards 1994).

During the first stage, also called the stage of mutual acquaintance, we usually observe a hierarchical organisational structure with a tendency towards an autocratic leadership, with friendly interactions between members but not getting too personal. Overall productivity of the team is usually low. This phase is often referred to as 'forming' or the state of a 'Basic Team' according to MacMillan (2001).

During the second stage, often described as the 'storming' stage, the team makes an effort to achieve a common goal. This phase can be characterised by the formation of alliances built on common interests. It might also lead to conflicts due to lack of clarity of the varied professionals' roles to be assumed. The use of different professional terms or jargons can also lead to misunderstandings between professionals from different backgrounds. This type of team is also referred to as an 'Adolescent Team' (MacMillan 2001).

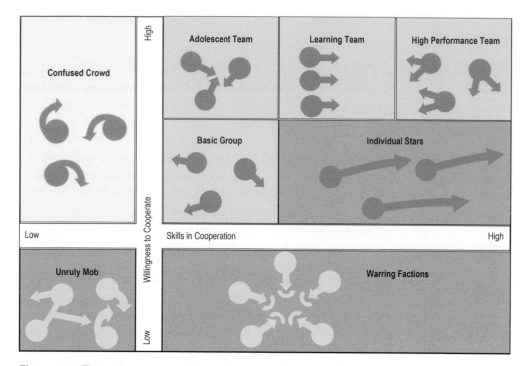

Figure 6.3 The various stages of team development can be described in terms of willingness to collaborate and skill in cooperation

After the 'storming' phase, the third stage is characterised by a degree of passivity due to the growing insecurity and indecision of the team members. On one hand the desire to achieve a common goal continues, but on the other hand the desire grows to avoid conflicts that could paralyse further actions. Members become aware that the interpretation of goals might be different and that there might be areas lacking mutual agreement or with different sets of values. This 'norming' stage raises the need for common norms and rules, leading to the fourth stage.

The fourth stage is also often denominated as the 'crisis' stage, and is characterised by members voicing their concerns and disagreements more openly and emotionally. Eventually the crisis can enable the team to come to agree on core principles and values.

The fifth stage, the 'resolution', requires open communication, shared leadership and transparency about decisions made.

Once these elements of the resolution are in place the team enters the sixth and final stage in this process, the stage of maintenance of the team or the stage of 'performing'. (Stages three, four and five are also seen as aspects of 'norming'.) In the performing stage the needs and values of the patients and clients have the highest priority, and the primary communication goals between team members are to attend to those needs. Teams in the 'norming' phase are described by MacMillan as 'Learning Teams'; those that are 'performing' would be called 'High-Performance Teams' (MacMillan 2001).

We all know what it is like to be a member of an effective high-performing team – and we also know what it is like to be a member of a team that is not effective. To ensure effective patient care and the delivery of systems for health, one of the things we need to do is try to ensure we have teams that are working well, and where we have teams that are not, to help them be more effective. In the Appendices readers can find further descriptions of the issues that can affect different types of teams and how skills and willingness to work in the team contribute to make them high-performing or dysfunctional (See Appendix 2).

Health professionals as 'environmental factors'

By asking for assistance, a person enlarges their 'environment' with the addition of professionals with whom they work. As is well recognised, the environment has an important impact on everybody's life; in this case, a positive impact is needed and wanted.

Professionals are expected to facilitate the problem resolution of the person with whom they are working. This means that professionals need to have a clear understanding of the issues of our patients as a starting point for our shared approach to addressing these issues. It is up to health professionals to ask the right questions, to listen and interpret carefully, and to share information. This will allow us both to get to know more about the things the person themself defines as a problem, and to help them be able to talk about possible goals. By providing information and talking about things that a person perceives problematic, health professionals can explore the goals the person is pursuing.

Goal setting is not a traditional approach in healthcare, so patients often need help to describe their goals. It may therefore be unusual for patients to ask health professionals for help and tell them about the goals they are pursuing. We believe that it should become a common practice for health professionals to question how they might facilitate both their patients' goal setting and their decision-making. It may therefore be helpful to review the approach to this process of shared goal setting. This important process can appear to be linear, whereas in reality it is transactional – changing with time and the evolving issues. For this reason, the elements of time and change/development are essential ingredients as goals are both shaped and revised.

Even when a goal may appear to be small, every step needs special attention. These small steps are often taken unconsciously and may not appear to be clearly separated. Highlighting their separation here, in the notes below, is intended to make them explicit and to stress the possibilities and challenges connected to them.

Sharing information

Patients need health professionals who are comfortable and able to talk about functioning perspectives and possibilities, to enable patients to understand their problem and their goals. Patients also need to be willing and empowered to talk to professionals as equals.

Mandate clarification

The second step is to ask people about their own goals: what are they hoping for? There is a difference between one's implicit knowledge (and indeed assumptions) about the problem and people's problem-solving possibilities; it is therefore essential to make issues explicit, especially people's personal goals, which need to be sufficiently clarified. Without this explicit process, health professionals can easily miss a person's goals concerning activity and participation and simply focus on their traditional health professional business, namely addressing issues concerning body function and structure. The following questions to patients can be helpful in searching for the goals:

- What would you describe as your main problem?

- How does this issue become noticeable in, and affect, your daily life?

- What do you expect from my profession and from me as a professional?

- How will your life be different if we resolve the problem, or at least address it effectively?

- What in your life should remain as it is now?

These questions could help health professionals to clarify both their expected mandate and whether they would agree with the goals set by the person. They should ask explicitly for more detailed information about the person's activities. An example from the field of childhood disability might illustrate how discussion and negotiation can help to bridge both a conceptual and technical gap that is common in our practice. Parents of a child with significant functional challenges in mobility or communication have as their goals that their child should/will walk and talk – goals that might be long term, or even unattainable in the literal sense of the words 'walk' or 'talk'. By reframing these goals to 'enhancing mobility' ('We want him to be able to explore independently') and 'enhancing communication' ('We want to know what's on his mind') we may be able to get on the same page regarding 'Activity' (function) and help parents recognise the potential for their child to achieve these goals, even if they do things differently from 'normal' (Rosenbaum & Gorter 2012).

This person-oriented approach does not lead to a loss of the profession-oriented perspective; rather, with this approach patients have more confidence and trust in their healthcare professionals, while empathic health professionals can recognise and value the individual and the effects an intervention may have on that person and their roles in life as an individual, as well as on their body. The goals concerning a person's health and functional status must be reviewed by health professionals both to assess their feasibility and, by elaborating a management plan, to determine next steps and necessary interventions.

Search for the appropriate team members to address goals
Through mandate clarification and the determination of next steps and interventions it becomes clear who else should join the team. Which professions, and what skills, are needed? Who can provide or find important information to pursue the goals? How can these professionals become part of the team? In the clinical example above, it is obvious that we will need professionals with technical experience in fitting of, provision of appropriate augmentative interventions, and training in the use of such as powered mobility and communication aids to exploit the best capacities of children with impaired abilities to do things in a fashion that may be different from usual but that can enable 'typical' achievements.

Capturing the situation/junction of knowledge
Health professionals have varied ways to increase their knowledge about a person's functioning, and these will differ across professions. Focusing on functioning means gathering information on all aspects of the person's life as outlined within elements of the ICF. Life is complex, and there are many areas of a person's life to discover and share with professionals. Gathering information means trying to follow the complexity and richness of a person's life. This includes knowing their preferences and their capacity as well as their current performance (which may be quite a bit different from their capacity). Identifying factors within person, task and environment that create the gap between capacity and performance helps us to recognise opportunities to be creatively helpful. Capturing the situation is based on the knowledge transfer among the person, the professionals, and the proxies. This can lead to everyone being overwhelmed with too much information, so it is essential to be clear on a person's priorities.

Shared interpretation of knowledge and the search for solutions
The knowledge gained from a patient and their significant others needs to be interpreted by the team: 'Now that we know [the patient], what does this mean for us to do?'

Professionals need to be ready both to accept responsibilities for specific goals, and to step back and trust their colleagues as appropriate if others have the requisite skills. This is of course the essence of teamwork. Professionals have to listen to, and to talk with, each other, discussing the information and drawing conclusions on how to proceed. Professionals and patients need to be able, on an equal footing, to debate even contentious issues in order to agree on common goals and the choice of methods to achieve them.

Coordinated action
Coordinated action means that everybody knows about the goals being pursued and the methods chosen to reach them. Every member of the team – including the patient and family – knows of the actions of the others.

Further considerations: hidden goals
Considering the ethical guidelines for the use of ICF one finds that the person,

> whose level of functioning is being classified (or the person's advocate) should have the opportunity to participate, and in particular to challenge or affirm the appropriateness of the category being used and the assessment *assigned* (WHO 2013, p. 10).

In addition, the information should be used 'to the greatest extend feasible, with the collaboration of individuals to enhance their choices and their control over their lives' (WHO 2013).

Health professionals are supposed to talk with their patients with honesty and humility, to listen to them carefully and work with them on an equal level. Unfortunately, in clinical practice the goals explicitly communicated with patients are sometimes not the only ones. There may also be some hidden professional goals that might be developed by supporting patients during their coping process. Examples might include thinking such as: 'This person needs to learn that this won't be possible'. We may be thinking of possible changes concerning the lifestyle or the environment of a person (for example, 'It would be better for [the patient] to have more assistance by their father', or 'It is too untidy at [the patient]'s home; they watch too much TV.') This issue of hidden assumptions (often unconscious biases) needs some further reflection, in order to consider: 'Could this approach actually reflect the way services are organised?', 'Do management expectations influence hidden goals of professionals?', 'Can the ICF help professionals and patients to identify goals and make them more transparent?'

Clinical practice is infinitely varied because the people we work with – the people who seek our advice and help – are infinitely varied! Even when we work in specialty areas (as do the authors of this book with our focus on childhood disability) it is essential that we personalise all our efforts, and not apply this or that thinking to 'people with cerebral palsy' or 'families of kids with autism'. Concepts such as 'health' and 'functioning' are fundamentally individual constructs, related to personal, social and cultural norms and values (Cassel 1982). In talking about goals, we are thinking about norms and values as well. And these can be similar or different among the many people involved in patient care. For this reason, thinking about hidden goals is also an issue of social and cultural norms and values concerning the functioning of a person.

References

Bronfenbrenner U, Ceci S (1994) Nature-nurture reconceptualized in developmental perspective: A bioecological model. *Psychol Rev* **101**(4): 568–586.

Canadian Interprofessional Health Collaborative (2010) *A National Interprofessional Competency Framework*. Vancouver: Canadian Interprofessional Health Collaborative, University of British Columbia.

Cassel E (1982) The nature of suffering and the goals of medicine. *New Engl J Med* **306**(11): 641–645.

Dufour ADP, Lucy SD (2010) Situating primary health care within the International Classification of Functioning Disability and Health: Enabling the Canadian Family Health Team initiative. *J Interprof Care* **24**: 666–677.

Hollenweger J (2010) MHADIE's matrix to analyse the functioning of education systems. *Disabil Rehabil* **32**(S1): S116–S124.

Hugo J, Couper I (2006) Teaching consultation skills using juggling as a metaphor. *SA Family Pract* **48**(5): 5–7.

Journal of Interprofessional Care (2017) Instructions for authors [online]. *J Interprof Care.* http://www.tandfonline.com/action/authorSubmission?show=instructions&journalCode=ijic20.

MacMillan P (2001) *The Performance Factor*. Nashville, Tennessee: B&H Publishing Group.

Robards MF (1994) The multidisciplinary team. In: Robards MF *Running a Team for Disabled Children and their Families*. London: Mac Keith Press, p. 113.

Rosenbaum P, Gorter JW (2012) The 'F-words' in childhood disability: I swear this is how we should think! *Child Care Health Dev* **38**(4): 457–463.

Snyman S, Von Pressentin KB, Clarke M (2015) International Classification of Functioning Disability and Health: catalyst for interprofessional education and collaborative practice. *J Interprof Care* **29**(4): 313–9.

Snyman S, van Zyl M, Müller J, Geldenhuys M (2016) International Classification of Functioning Disability and Health: Catalyst for interprofessional education and collaborative practice. In: Forman D, Jones M, Thistlethwaite J (eds.) *Leading Research and Evaluation in Interprofessional Education and Collaborative Practice*. London: Palgrave Macmillan, pp. 285–328.

Sohns A (2000) Rechtliche Grundlagen der Frühförderung. *Frühförderung Interdisziplinär* **19**: 63–79.

Speck O (1996) Frühförderungentwicklungsauffalliger Kinder unter okologisch-integrativen Aspekt [Early intervention of children with developmental issues under ecological and integrative aspects]. In: Peterander F, Speck O (eds.) *Frühförderungin Europa*. Munich: Reinhardt Verlag.

Thurmair M, Naggl M (2000) *Praxis der Frühförderung*. München: Reinhardt.

Winiarski MG (1997) Understanding HIV/AIDS using the biopsychosocial/spiritual model. In: Winiarski MG (ed.) *HIV Mental Health for the 21st Century*. New York: New York University Press, pp. 3–22.

WHO (World Health Organization) (2007) *International Classification of Functioning Disability and Health: Children & Youth Version: ICF-CY*. Geneva: World Health Organization.

WHO (World Health Organization) (2013) *How to Use the ICF: A Practical Manual for Using the International Classification of Functioning Disability and Health (ICF)*. Geneva: World Health Organization.

Chapter 7

The ICF: Themes and tools for the education of health professionals

Olaf Kraus de Camargo and Stefanus Snyman

Background

The 1960s and 1970s marked a change of thinking in health and social care. In the field of social work Florence Hollis coined the term 'person-in-situation' (Cornell 2006) and in developmental psychology, Bronfenbrenner is well known for his ecological model of human development, also first proposed in the 1970s (Bronfenbrenner & Morris 2007). In medicine, George Engel identified the need for 'a new model in medicine', introducing the term 'bio-psycho-social model' (Engel 1977) which eventually informed the development of the ICF. The zeitgeist of the 1970s influenced the discussion about how future health professionals should be educated, and the voices calling for change increased. Williams (1974) wrote:

> The medical schools have failed to teach students and doctors the comprehensive approach to medicine, and that the sciences of sociology and psychology are equal in importance to physiology, biochemistry and anatomy, and that the practice of community medicine and prevention is as important as hospital medicine.

Such dissatisfaction led to innovative ways to teach medicine, with the introduction of problem-based learning (PBL) as pioneered at McMaster University. In an article from 1975 introducing the program Sweeney and Mitchell (1975) describe its goals:

> The MD graduate is expected to identify, define, and solve problems related to human health by examining the underlying biological, social, and behavioural mechanisms involved. … By using this technique, it is hoped that the students are

made aware of the complex and challenging problems of man as an individual within society before they are wooed by the intellectually intriguing problems in structure and function of man's component parts.

Despite those early indications of a need for change, today's health educators continue to struggle to form and shape professionals who are attuned to the needs of the population. The statements at an academic event at the Stanford Medicine X conference 'Reimagining Health Care Education' exemplify this:

> 'health care has become so complex. Skills are so specialized. Collaboration is not a nice-to-have, it's a must-have. And therefore, we're moving toward team-based approaches.'

> 'Interprofessional, interdisciplinary, team-based collaboration is essential to the future of our functioning health care system. And we can't get there if we're not learning and teaching together.'

> 'Lastly, we're shifting the model because there's a whole generation of new tools – digital health, data that's coming in and empowering the end user to take control and to be more collaborative. And we're realizing that costs have become so out of control that the old model of paternalistic medicine, of hierarchal medicine, is unsustainable. It doesn't work. We have to create a model of engagement where people want to participate, and want to engage, so that there's buy-in and personal responsibility' (James 2017).

The statements from the 1970s – and contemporary echoes of these ideas – emphasise the importance of communication between clinicians and patients, the importance of recognising the influence of contextual factors to health, and the importance of patients and health professionals learning with, for and from one another using the same language.

These developments have been explained by Frenk et al. (2010) as three generations of health education reforms, of which we have witnessed two. The first occurred at the beginning of the 20th century with the introduction of a science-based curriculum; in the mid-20th century the second reform was characterised by the implementation of problem-based learning. The next reform will need to address not only the training of health professionals in how to be able to better collaborate, but also will require an improvement of the performance of healthcare systems (Frenk et al. 2010).

Health professional education and the role of the ICF

There is global consensus that the vision of health professional education (HPE) is to achieve health equity (WHO 2010, 2014, Frenk et al. 2010, Global Consensus for Social Accountability in Medical Schools 2010). Frenk et al. (2010) argued that huge strides in achieving health equity could be made if a person/patient-centred approach to education (as opposed to the current primarily biomedical approach) were adopted, and if students were trained in communities (and thus had population-based experiences and not the heavy emphasis on tertiary institution-based exposures).

Figure 7.1 (adapted from Frenk et al. 2010) illustrates that the instructional (educational) reforms that are needed to achieve health equity should focus on transformative learning, equipping students and professionals as agents of change with the competencies needed to function in communities and demonstrating person- and community-centredness.

Transforming HPE by adopting person-centredness requires competencies related to biopsychosocial-spiritual approaches to health, incorporating the complex interrelatedness of (1) changes in body functions and body structures, (2) functioning and fulfilling life roles, in the context of (3) barriers and facilitators of environmental factors influencing health (including social determinants of health) and (4) personal factors influencing health. This transformed approach should result in holistic care, shared decision-making and person-reported outcomes, creating the opportunity for person-driven data (Snyman et al. 2015).

The institutional (organisational) reform needed to achieve health equity alludes to greater interdependence between higher education training institutions and service providers (i.e. universities and departments of health) in bridging the huge gap that often exists between the two systems.

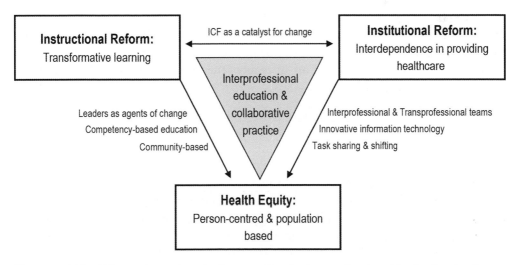

Figure 7.1 The ICF can play a pivotal role as catalyst for instructional and institutional reforms needed in health professions education for reaching health equity
Adapted from Frenk et al. (2010)

Reforming systems for health requires a focus on community-based practice through harmonising health education (interdependence), by breaking down silos and professional tribalism, embracing interprofessional and transprofessional collaborative practice, task shifting, task sharing, decreasing power relations and innovatively using information technology. These are necessary if we are to provide universal health coverage by reducing institutionalised care, focusing on preventive healthcare, ultimately resulting in predictive healthcare. The latter is dependent on big data, obtained by utilising paradigm-shifting person-driven data sources (Snyman et al. 2015).

Those using the ICF in practice will likely agree with Snyman, von Pressentin and Clarke (2015) that introducing the ICF into health professional education has the potential to support the third reform proposed by Frenk (Snyman et al. 2015). The framework of the ICF can add the necessary biopsychosocial-spiritual approach, allowing us to capture more effectively the social dimensions and the personal perspectives of people with health conditions. The ICF provides a common language for all professionals and patients/caregivers, and can ultimately be used to collect data about the functional health of populations. By these means the ICF can support necessary institutional transformation and reforms, and eventually contribute to greater health equity by providing care to people based on their individual needs (Snyman et al. 2015).

Examples of ICF education

A conceptual paper by Stephenson and Richardson proposed the ICF as a common framework in health education to facilitate the necessary paradigm shift for healthcare in the 21st century (Stephenson & Richardson 2008). In a review article by Bornbaum et al. (2014) the authors reflected on 10 years of literature and found 18 publications related to the topic. They state:

> Indeed, it is likely that health professionals well trained in the ICF are best positioned to move ICF values about functioning and disability forward by engaging the general public at large and facilitating the culture change we seek.

One way this change might happen is through a top-down approach by different professional organisations endorsing the use of the ICF in the training of their professionals, as has already been done by the American Speech–Language–Hearing Association, the American Physical Therapy Association, the Canadian Institute for Health Information and the Institute of Medicine in North America (Bornbaum et al. 2014). Examples from Europe include the International Bobath Association (IBITA 2016) and the German Association for Social Paediatrics and Adolescent Medicine (DGSPJ 2014). In Latin America, the Brazilian Federal Council for Physiotherapy and Occupational

Therapy (COFFITO) endorses the ICF to its members and launched a free online course for its members in 2016 (COFFITO 2016). These endorsements are in accordance with WHO recommendations to use the ICF 'in curriculum design and to raise awareness and undertake social action'.

While endorsements are positive, they do not necessarily lead to concrete steps towards implementation. It is therefore interesting to review examples where this has been done, in the hope to learn from those experiences, as described below.

Germany
One of the first formal accounts of including the ICF as part of the curriculum in health professional education comes from the German Society of Rehabilitation Science and the German Society for Physical Medicine and Rehabilitation in 2004. They proposed a new interprofessional course to be included in the revision of the federal medical training regulations called 'Rehabilitation, Physical Medicine, Naturopathic Treatment', and the ICF was to be a fundamental part in this course (Mau et al. 2004). In their arguments for including the ICF the authors state:

> The education of health professionals should also include emotional objectives to understand changes of values and priorities of people along life and life experiences, contributing to a positive, activating attitude towards people with disabilities in an environment of mostly acute care and curative approaches to disease. … This requires preparedness to work collaboratively with other health professionals.

The Hannover Medical School later adapted these ideas and started teaching ICF concepts in what became known as the 'Hannover Model' (Gutenbrunner et al. 2010). A major limitation in these early models of teaching the ICF is that they were often still directed to one single group of healthcare workers (MDs) (whereas the ICF is meant to be used across professions and disciplines); even within that course of Medicine, the exposure is restricted to the field of rehabilitation. Not having other professions and disciplines being taught the ICF makes it difficult to implement it into interprofessional clinical practice. It also conveys the (wrong) impression that the ICF has a boutique niche in 'rehab medicine' rather than universal applicability.

Another example from Germany are the curricula of Early Childhood Intervention courses (BA) at some Universities for Applied Sciences (FH Nordhausen, Medical School Hamburg – the first a public institution and the latter a private organisation). Those curricula were developed from workshops for continuing professional education (with more than 500 participants over the years); were practice oriented; and were geared towards the interprofessional teams working in German Early Childhood Intervention Centres as well as Social Paediatric Centres. The approach of these courses is to stimulate discussion in small groups of learners, using the ICF to better describe and understand people with different impairments. The ICF is used as a tool to address all relevant aspects in the life of a person and, based on this analysis, to develop plans for supports and intervention. Many of the materials in this current book have been used during those workshops and in the curricula of the courses referenced.

The Netherlands

Academics of the program of Occupational Epidemiology at Maastricht University, the Research Centre for Rehabilitation, Work and Sports at the University of Applied Sciences in Nijmegen and the Department of Medical Humanities at the VU University Medical Centre in Amsterdam developed a curriculum for their students entitled *Occupational Health from a Biopsychosocial Perspective: an Evidence Based Approach* (de Brouwer et al. 2015). This curriculum includes teaching the ICF as a common language, ICF linking rules, developing ICF core sets and use of the ICF in Monitoring and Surveillance. In addition, the authors gave consideration to the fact that students coming from a biomedical learning environment will require additional skills to be able to work with a biopsychosocial model of health. They added to the course a second part dedicated to teaching critical appraisal of evidence under the lens of the ICF and preparing students to work clinically within a biopsychosocial framework, engaging with their clients on a holistic level.

Alberta, Canada

At the University of Alberta, the ICF was one of the guiding principles when redesigning the curriculum for Physiotherapy. The department wanted the curriculum to integrate the philosophy and language of the ICF, valorising the importance of person-centred practice, based on evidence and a good understanding of theoretical frameworks (Darrah et al. 2006). The interaction between theory, research and clinical practice and its relation to the ICF framework is described in the Clinical Decision-Making Model in Figure 7.2 (Darrah et al. 2006).

This is an example of very thoughtful implementation, making all the connections between the framework necessary to organise ideas and the practical implications in both research and clinical practice. It focuses less on 'finding the right code' than on the conceptual connectedness of issues.

Ontario, Canada

The School of Rehabilitation Science at McMaster University offers an elective course about the ICF open to students from any field in the university. The course is organised into introductory lectures followed by individual projects developed by the students and supervised by faculty mentors. With that approach, the goal is directed towards students acquiring a good understanding of the framework and potential applications of the ICF in research, administration and clinical practice. Some of the projects initiated during the course have been developed further and resulted in publications (Nguyen et al. 2016).

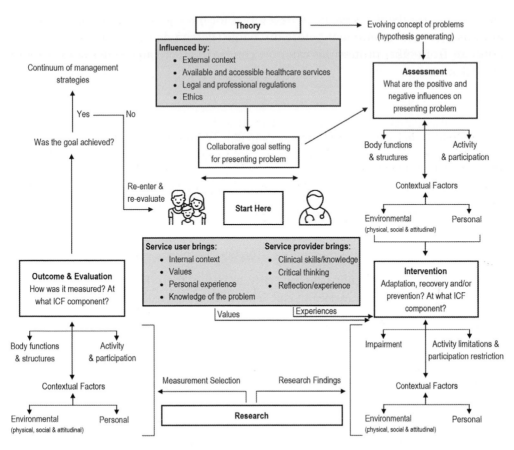

Figure 7.2 The C.O.R.E Clinical Decision-making model
Darrah et al. 2006. Reprinted with permission from Taylor and Francis.
Icons made by Freepik and Prosymbols from www.flaticon.com

Brazil

The endorsement of the ICF by the Brazilian Association of Physiotherapy and Occupational Therapy and the inclusion of the ICF as part of new disability laws in that country has generated a great demand for education about the ICF. The organisation CIFBrasil (ICF Brazil) offers both online and offline courses (face-to-face contact sessions) for professionals and has presented those courses in all states of Brazil. Together with the online modules, over 9000 professionals have received training in the ICF to date (Santana Cordeiro 2015). Some municipalities have started to adopt the ICF as part of the documentation of the health status of the population in primary care (Santana Cordeiro & Carlos de Oliveira Júnior 2014).

At the Federal University of Sergipe, in the Brazilian Northeast Region, the University Hospital has been adopting the ICF for teaching of students of physiotherapy.

Tools based on the ICF have been developed for managing triage in orthopaedics and to assess goal attainment before discharge (Pereira de Farias Neto et al. 2017). Students from other professions can now choose to attend an elective course about the ICF at that university.

Chile

In Chile, the dissemination of the ICF started with one physiotherapist (Daniel Cid) at Talca University. Initially, the courses were part of a master's project in case management of children with physical disabilities (Cid Cofre 2011), but now several further education courses are being offered, for both clinical and administrative purposes (Cid Cofre 2016). So far about 150 professionals have been trained. In 2017, the concept of the ICF has been included in a postgraduate course at the Faculty of Medicine at the University of Chile (University of Chile 2017).

South Africa

Medical students at Stellenbosch University, as part of their decentralised rotation in Family Medicine, Community Health and Rehabilitation, are required to manage patients interprofessionally using an ICF frame of reference. In the process, they need to engage students from other health services professions, or relevant health or social care professionals, to manage patients from a biopsychosocial-spiritual perspective. The holistic assessment also includes a home and/or work visit to evaluate performance and contextual factors. At the end of the rotation students have to present the actions taken or orchestrated by them to an interprofessional team of preceptors from the local health facility. Initially these professionals, with the occasional exception, didn't know a thing about ICF, although the rubric they used to assess the students was based on the ICF. Within 2 to 3 months the Interprofessional Education team at Stellenbosch University received various requests from health professionals at these facilities to be trained in how to use the ICF in the holistic management of patients. The professionals' motivation was their impression that the patients managed by students received better care. They realised that patients' problems were addressed holistically, that longstanding issues were resolved, that continuity of care improved and that fewer patients were 'recycled' through the system (Snyman, Von Pressentin and Clarke 2015).

One professor, referring to medical students in their second year of clinical rotations, stated that he had 'never experienced such a holistic and thorough management of patients, not even by Family Medicine residents'. One patient stated that 'doctors will be more useful … if they ask me the questions these students did'. However, the perception was reported that 'once you are a doctor you just run through things, but these students thought broader'.

Subsequently, a very elementary three-session course was developed to fit into the weekly journal of mortality and morbidity meetings at these health facilities (Table 7.1).

Table 7.1 Outline of the elementary ICF course

Day 1

SESSION 1 (Contact Session)

2 Hours (Including 15 Minutes Ethics/Human Rights)

Before first session: Reflection 1 (100 words: who are you; why are you here; what do you know of ICF; what are your expectations)

Introductions

Introduction to health professions education for 21st century: Strategy of Faculty of health sciences

Overview of the ICF framework in the context of ethics and human rights

Interprofessional teams work out and present a case study based on ICF framework

After day 1 and before next contact session (group work)

4 hours (incl 30 minutes ethics/human rights)

Structured reflection (hand-outs on reflection) (1h).

Interprofessional teams prepare one patient to present (3h, including ethics/human rights 30 minutes)

Day 2

SESSION 3 (Contact Session)

2 hours (incl 15 minutes ethics/human rights)

Feedback from group and facilitators

Presentation and discussions of real case studies by interprofessional teams. Summative and formative peer-assessment and interrater validation (including ethics/human rights 15 minutes)

Discussion on the road ahead and preparation for the next contact day

SESSION 4 (Group work)

1 hour (incl 10 minutes ethics/human rights)

Summative and formative assessment of student presentation (including ethics/human rights 10 minutes)

After day 2 and before next contact session (group work)

4 hours (incl 30 minutes ethics/human rights)

Structured reflection on interprofessional case discussions and your own interprofessional practice. (1 hour)

Interprofessional team conducts literature study and prepares a draft document to submit to superiors motivating the ICF approach to encourage interprofessional patient-centred care. (4 hours)

(Continued)

Table 7.1 (Continued)

Day 3
SESSION 5 (Group work)
2 hours (incl 10 minutes ethics/human rights)
Interprofessional groups conduct a ward round/case discussion in hospital (1 patient for a group) based on ICF framework, including team discussion, management plan and shared decision-making with the patient (Ethics/Human rights: 10 minutes)
Discussion and formative feedback
Feedback by interprofessional teams regarding their proposed approach to present to your superiors a motivation to promote the use of the ICF framework to improve patient- and community-centred care (Ethics/Human rights: 10 minutes).
After Day 3 (Own Time)
Evaluation of course

http://icfeducation.org/resources/99.

A year later these health professionals and students reported that they took the application of ICF a step further. Initially an ICF framework, printed on an A3-size piece of paper, found its way to over-bed trolleys, where everyone on the team summarised their findings. This served as the basis for interprofessional communication for when professionals were not able to meet face-to-face, for priority setting, and for shared decision-making. Five years down the line this form has matured and now forms part of the official stationery of the Western Cape Government (see Appendix 4).

But the story didn't stop here. The paper system had serious shortcomings. In the rural districts members of interprofessional teams have huge geographical areas to cover and are seldom together at the same place to assess patients together or to attend interprofessional case discussions. Furthermore, it is not optimal to ensure continuity of care by copying forms and sending them back and forth. Subsequently, students and professionals requested a patient-driven mHealth application to allow patients to record and share their own 'ICF profile' with their health professionals, also allowing professionals to add their contributions. The same need was identified in Canada by Olaf Kraus de Camargo of *CanChild at McMaster University. This gave birth to the development of the* **ICanFunction mHealth Solution** *(mICF) with over 20 partners globally collaborating on this innovative project* (www.icfmobile.org).

In this interprofessional education process in South Africa, the ICF sold itself. Students served as change agents and the ICF as the catalyst for an interprofessional biopsychosocial-spiritual approach to care. For their part, the health professionals who began using and teaching ICF as early adopters advocated for the ICF with their superiors and healthcare administrators.

Conclusion

We find increasing evidence of a variety of approaches to people teaching and applying the ICF. These approaches differ with regard to the target population (undergraduate, graduate, postgraduate, continuing professional development) and the focus (teaching the framework, integrating the framework into clinical practice and research, learning how to code). In many instances, these initiatives build on the passion of early adopters and pioneers, striving to change (and improve) the way we provide healthcare, sharing common values of collaborative practice and patient-centred/driven care. Until the ICF is a standard part of curricula it will be necessary to continue with different approaches, and to learn from all of them. The endorsement through professional organisations is a helpful first step and can facilitate the dissemination of ICF knowledge among practicing professionals, as is occurring in Brazil. The fundamental goals of teaching the ICF should be to create awareness of the framework and use of the 'ICF language' in communication about, and with persons, using health services. The details of coding can be relevant for research (linking different assessment tools) and gathering functional health information. However, just as drilling vocabulary lists should not be the approach to learning a new language, in the opinion of the authors the ICF codes should not be the focus of teaching.

References

Boelen C (2010) Global consensus on social accountability of medical schools. Sante Publique. **23**(3): 247–250.

Bornbaum CC, Day AMB, Izaryk K, et al. (2014) Exploring use of the ICF in health education. *Disabil Rehabil* **37**(2): 179–186.

Bronfenbrenner U, Morris PA (2007) The Bioecological Model of Human Development. In: Damon W, Lerner R, editors. *Handbook of Child Psychology*. Hoboken, NJ, USA: John Wiley & Sons, Inc.; pp. 795–828.

Cid Cofre DE (2011) *Proposition of a Collaboration Node between Health and Education Services for Preeschoolers with Physical Disabilities* [*Propuesta de Nodo Salud / Educación para Pre-escolares con Discapacidad Física*]. Talca: Universidad de Talca.

Cid Cofre DE (2016) Centro de Innovacion e Desarollo en Ambitos de Salud – CIDEAS [online]. http://cideas.cl/web/.

COFFITO. COFFITO lança plataforma de Ensino a Distância e oferece curso sobre CIF aos profissionais [Internet]. 2016 [cited 2017 Jul 28]. Available from: https://www.coffito.gov.br/nsite/?p=5324.

Cornell KL (2006) Person-in-situation: history theory and new directions for social work practice. *PRAXIS* **6**: 50–57.

Damon W, Lerner R (eds.) Handbook of Child Psychology. Hoboken, NJ: John Wiley & Sons, pp. 795–828.

Darrah J, Loomis J, Manns P, Norton B, May L (2006) Role of conceptual models in a physical therapy curriculum: application of an integrated model of theory research and clinical practice. *Physiother Theory Pract* **22**(5): 239–250.

de Brouwer CPM, Heerkens YF, Kant IJ (eds.) (2015) Occupational Health from a Biopsychosocial perspective – an Evidence Based Approach. Maastricht: Mediview BV.

DGSPJ (Deutsche Gesellschaft fur Sozialpadiatrie und Jugendmedizin e.V.) (2002) *Altöttinger Papier Beitrag zur Qualitätssicherung in Sozialpädiatrischen Zentren.* Altotting: Deutsche Gesellschaft fur Sozialpadiatrie und Jugendmedizin e.V.

DGSPJ (2014) Checklisten ICF-CY [online]. *Deutsche Gesellschaft fur Sozialpadiatrie und Jugenmedizin.* http://www.dgspj.de/service/icf-cy/.

Engel GL (1977) The need for a new medical model: a challenge for biomedicine. *Science* **196**(4286): 129–136.

Frenk J, Chen L, Bhutta ZA, et al. (2010) Health professionals for a new century: transforming education to strengthen health systems in an interdependent world. *Lancet* **376**: 1923–1958.

Gutenbrunner C, Schiller J, Schwarze M, et al. (2010) Hannover model for the implementation of physical and rehabilitation medicine teaching in undergraduate medical training. *J Rehabil Med* **42**(3): 206–213.

IBITA (International Bobath Instructors Training). *Core Curriculum for the Basic Course on the Evaluation and Treatment of Adults with Neurological Conditions - The Bobath Concept [Internet].* International Bobath Instructors Training Association - IBITA; 2016 [cited 2018 Oct 21]. p. 8. Available from: https://ibita.org/basic-course/.

James J (2017) Reimagining health care education – Stanford Medicine X [online]. https://medicinex.stanford.edu/2017/04/17/reimagining-health-care-education/.

Mau W, Gülich M, Gutenbrunner C, et al. (2004) Lernziele im querschnittsbereich Rehabilitation Physikalische Medizin und Naturheilverfahren nach der 9. Revision der Approbationsordnung für Ärzte: Gemeinsame empfehlung der Deutschen Gesellschaft für Rehabilitations-wissenschaften und der Deutschen Ges. *Physikalische Medizin Rehabilitationsmedizin Kurortmedizin* **14**(6): 308–318.

Nguyen T, Fayed N, Gorter JW, MacDermid J (2016) Enhancing interprofessional education and practice: Development and implementation of a new graduate-level course using the International Classification of Functioning Disability and Health. *J Interprof Care* **1820**: 1–3.

Pereira de Farias Neto J, Uruga Oliveira G, Salgueiro Santana MM, et al. (2017) Experiência Prática Da Universidade Federal De Sergipe/Hospital Universitário: Inclusão do Modelo Biopsicosocial e da CIF [Experience at the Federal University of Sergipe/University Hospital: Inclusion of the Biopsicosocial Model and ICF]. In: Santana Cordeiro E,Biz MCP (eds.) *Implantando a CIF: o que acontece na prática? [Implementing ICF: What happens in practice?].* Rio de Janeiro: WAK 292.

Santana Cordeiro E (2015) ICF online training for Brazilian professionals. *First International Symposium: ICF Education.* Helsinki, Finland.

Santana Cordeiro E, Carlos de Oliveira Júnior J (2014) A Aplicação Da Cif Por Agentes Comunitários De Saúde [The ICF application by health community agents]. *Revista Cientifica CIFBrasil* **1**(1): 18–26.

Snyman S, Anttila H, Kraus de Camargo O (2015) ICF Education: Rationale. *First International Symposium: ICF Education.* Helsinki Finland.

Snyman S, Von Pressentin KB, Clarke M (2015) International Classification of Functioning Disability and Health: catalyst for interprofessional education and collaborative practice. *J Interprof Care* **29**(4): 313–9.

Stephenson R, Richardson B (2008) Building an interprofessional curriculum framework for health: A paradigm for health function. *Adv Health Sci Edu* **13**(4): 547–557.

Sweeney GD, Mitchell DLM (1975) An introduction to the study of medicine: Phase I of the McMaster MD. Program. *J Med Edu* **50:** 70–77.

University of Chile (2017) 'Diploma for Assessment and Treatment of People with Neurologic Conditions' Neurofunctional Concept ['Diploma para la Valoración y tratamiento de personas en condiciones neurológicas'. Concepto Neurofuncional] [online]. http://www.medicina. uchile.cl/cursos/131028/diploma-para-la-valoracion-y-tratamiento-de-personas.

Williams H (1974) Perspectives in medical practice and education. *Aust Paediatr J* **10**(Suppl. 3): 32–34.

WHO (World Health Organization) (2010) Framework for action on interprofessional education and collaborative practice [Internet]. Geneva: World Health Organization. http://www.who. int/hrh/nursing_midwifery/en/.

WHO (World Health Organization) (2014) WHO global disability action plan 2014–2021: Better health for all people with disability [Internet]. Geneva: World Health Organization.

Chapter 8

The ICF informing administration, policy and advocacy

Olaf Kraus de Camargo and Jaclyn Pederson

ICF also serves as a potentially powerful tool for evidence-based advocacy. It provides reliable and comparable data to make the case for change. The political notion that disability is as much the result of environmental barriers as it is of health conditions or impairments must be transformed, first into a research agenda and then into valid and reliable evidence. This evidence can bring genuine social change for persons with disabilities around the world. (WHO 2007, p. 256).

Administrative applications

To be able to fulfil its mandate the WHO requires population-based data. This was the impulse that led to the development of different classification systems (examples include the regularly-updated ICD series, the ICF and ICF-CY, and a host of disease-specific classifications [e.g. myeloid neoplasms (Vardiman et al. 2002)]) to allow people to structure and organise such data. Those systems are part of WHO's 'Family of International Classifications' (WHO-FIC), of which the ICF is a member. When the ICF was developed, it had to respect certain organisational rules and hierarchies, called a taxonomy (WHO 2007). The term 'taxonomy' is also used in other classifications; for example, the classification of the living species in biology. For animals we classify the 'classes' of amphibians, reptiles, birds and mammals under the topic 'Terrestrial, vertebrate animals'. In the ICF the first number of each item indicates the chapter in which it belongs; the letters before the code indicate the component (a higher level) to which the item belongs.

This structure allows people to use the ICF to describe the health status of a patient across several 'dimensions' of their health condition, at different levels and in different degrees of granularity. It also facilitates the use of aggregated data at the level of an institution. For example, the ICF can be used to answer questions such as: 'What are the most common barriers our clients encounter?', 'What type of support is most frequently necessary?', 'What types of professional skills are most commonly required?' Discussing the difficulties of using the ICF in such a broad application (as the system is currently developed), Wolfgang Cibis points out that:

> it lacks the operationalisation of the degrees of severity, the personal factors have not been developed, a systematic coding is not only time-consuming and difficult but the purpose of doing it is not clear. The massive collection of data to analyse the individual situation of a rehabilitation patient needs to be weighed against the right of each person to protection of personal data (Cibis 2009, p. 6).

When planning to collect and analyse personal data it is necessary to protect the patient's privacy (Deutsches Institut für Jugendhilfe und Familienrecht (DIJuF) e.V., 2015). To ensure this, data collection should only occur with the active participation of the individual. (Of course, doing so also adds the true 'voice' of the patient and not simply the professionals' perspectives.) Patients and families need to be informed and provide consent for the purpose of the collection and possible transmission of the data. The appendix of the ICF contains ethical guidelines for such a use of the classification (WHO 2007). It states that the description of the health status using the ICF should not result in any disadvantage for the patient.

Nonetheless, there is an ongoing discussion in the scientific literature arguing in favour of creating content for personal factors and using them in clinical practice. In Germany, such positions are promoted by the medical services of the health insurance companies (MDK). The goal is to:

> sensitise social physicians [as the physicians that approve claims are called] to the importance of personal factors in their task of evaluating patients, to understand their individual situation in all relevant dimensions and perform a goal-oriented assessment (Grotkamp et al. 2010).

In their 2010 paper, Grotkamp et al. stress the importance of the idea that the proposed personal factors should not be used in a discriminatory way. This good intention is laudable, but the process of an 'external' assessment and therefore a judgment outside of a physician–patient relationship may risk leading eventually to discrimination, to the extent that it is based on unchangeable personal characteristics (for example, religion, ethnicity, sex or age). During a professional consultation that is initiated by the patient, a trusting relationship is established, and for that relationship to be useful the knowledge and awareness of personal factors is of the utmost importance. This information is gathered through conversations with the patient assessing their goals, needs and motivation, but it is not necessary for that information to be collected or shared outside of that relationship. In opposition to this clinical importance of personal factors, the question has also been raised as to whether they are indeed necessary in terms of a classification or if they need better definitions to continue to be part of the classification (Simeonsson et al. 2014, Leonardi et al. 2015). (See Chapter 3 for a more detailed discussion.)

Several examples that describe the analysis of services that use the ICF-CY can be found in the literature. Frequently they are focused on a certain aspect of care (e.g. family-centredness [Darrah et al. 2012]) or the functional health of a specific population (e.g. children with cerebral palsy in Thailand [Tantilipikorn et al. 2012]). Those publications present ICF data that were generated a posteriori by analysing the existing documentation and then mapping it to ICF items. The difficulty in using such a procedure occurs when, in addition to the codes, the qualifiers for severity are also used. Deciding about a qualifier based on clinical descriptions can be quite subjective and lead to errors or distortions. By definition, an ICF qualifier is presented as a percentage of a limitation of functioning in any of the components. Without having been criterion-referenced and validated with a measurement tool using modern principles of measurement development, such qualifiers continue to be subjective and are not known to be either reliable (used consistently) or valid (clinically meaningful). This is one of the main barriers for a broader acceptance of the ICF as a documentation or classification tool.

In our experience we had the same concerns and therefore decided to use only a dichotomous coding scheme, as first suggested by Simeonsson & Lollar (2006), to develop an 'ICF-CY Checklist' for Early Intervention Centres in Germany. In a pilot study in two centres we assessed the frequency of the chosen goals by the teams using this checklist (Kraus de Camargo et al. 2007). To our surprise, we found that most goals selected by the therapists and early childhood educators were from the component of body functions and only a small number related to the areas of participation and environmental factors. This result allowed the teams to reflect on their approach and to discuss how they might improve the participation of children with disabilities and their families. A similar observation was made by Johanna Darrah and colleagues in Alberta, Canada when they assessed the family-centredness of children's treatment centres. While all the managers were convinced that family-centredness was a central aspect of their approach, the actual data indicated that frequently this was not the case. This shows the benefits of assessing the work done at an institutional level, using a common framework, and then reflecting on the results obtained (Darrah et al. 2012).

Another use of the ICF in institutions can be for internal team development purposes. Team members can use the ICF to describe their own areas of competence and action. This can be used to visualise core competencies, overlaps, gaps and highly specialised competencies that can only be offered by a few expert members. For managers, it is more meaningful to have such an overview than a list of professions to plan further competency building (Kraus de Camargo & Fayed 2013).

In cases in which institutions decide to implement a continuous quality improvement process,the ICF can provide indicators as a basis to choose outcome criteria and adequate tools to measure those (Kertoy et al. 2013).

Using the ICF-CY can be a good foundation for implementing a regular assessment of one's own practice. The modified and simplified ICF-CY lists (known as code sets), as developed, for example, by the German interdisciplinary working group as an adaptation of the ICF (Deutsche Interdisziplinäre Arbeitsgruppe zur ICF Adaptation für den Kinder- und Jugendbereich 2012, see downloadable English version http://www.mackeith.co.uk/ shop/icf-a-hands-on-approach-for-clinicians-and-families/), offer the opportunity to use the codes in the ICF for different purposes. The added attribute 'I' (Information) after an item indicates that this is an area of functioning that requires more assessments or collection of additional information from other sources. The attribute 'F' (*Förderung* – German for 'Intervention/Support') indicates an area chosen for a goal for intervention. Having such a system in place at the institutional level makes it possible to generate information about certain needs. For example, if it is noted that a significant number of patients are identified as requiring more information about their hearing level, a decision can be made to modify the referral process or to advocate implementing audiology services in the centre. Analysing the selected goals can, in this way, provide information about the competencies required among the staff and whether special training,or hiring staff with specific competencies, is indicated. At a community level, such information can be used to identify resource gaps.

At a regional level, similar possibilities of analysis exist if data from different institutions are anonymised and shared. Such an analysis would compile not only a list of diagnoses and conditions in the area but also indicate the most common barriers encountered. With regards to funding streams, it might also be more useful to determine the needs of a population or a group of people based on their functional needs than based on diagnostic categories. The latter approach, too frequently used, easily leads to discrimination, often because some diagnostic groups have a strong lobby to advocate for funding that then is limited to people within that diagnostic group; at times the diagnosis is too rare and does not have any lobby at all (McDowell & O'Keeffe 2012). In addition, people with more complex manifestations of most conditions are over-represented in patient populations and lead professionals to acquire a biased experience of those conditions.

Advocacy applications

Categorical (diagnosis-specific) approaches to health issues ignore the reality that thinking at a functional level – across disorders, using a so-called non-categorical approach – allows people to see the commonalities across conditions that provide support for resources and services that can address the needs of the many rather the few. Thus, while the ICF can be useful in identifying needs by collecting and aggregating information from top-down at different levels, it can also serve those who actively want to share relevant information about how their health is affected in a bottom-up process to advocate for meaningful changes in policy and service development. Most advocacy groups are organised around a specific diagnosis. Children with diverse diagnoses affecting their development often share common functional limitations. Bundling forces and numbers around these issues rather than these diagnoses might be more effective than dividing the voice of the advocates into many separate (often quite small) groups as too often still happens.

One useful example of an area where families are affected by diverse diagnoses but share a common functional problem or challenge is the group called Feeding Matters (https://www.feedingmatters.org), which was set up by Shannon and Bob Goldwater.

When Shannon and Bob Goldwater's newborn triplets struggled to eat, they experienced first-hand the challenges faced by thousands of families each year. Born 14-weeks early, and each weighing a little over one pound, the triplets spent the first four months of their lives in the neonatal intensive care unit (NICU). Once each baby was released, Shannon and Bob quickly realised feeding their children would become the greatest struggle for their young family of five. Each child struggled to eat, and all would choke, cough, and gag during mealtimes.

The Goldwater family founded 'Feeding Matters' in 2006 to help children with feeding disorders and create a support system for families. The organisation focuses on education, advocacy, research, early identification, collaborative care, and support for families that have children with paediatric feeding disorders and the healthcare professionals who care for them.

A paediatric feeding disorder is defined as a severe disruption to eating, drinking, or digestion that may cause medical problems and compromise growth and development. Currently, paediatric feeding disorders are treated as a symptom and do not have their own identity. Yet, paediatric feeding disorders affect more than 1 million children in the United States with over 200 diagnoses putting children at a higher risk for a paediatric feeding disorder. Due to this, Shannon Goldwater envisioned a time when healthcare professionals and families alike would have an identifiable name for paediatric feeding disorders – with a clear definition and individual diagnostic code. This vision led 'Feeding Matters' to host a consensus conference in March 2016 with 19 individuals representing multiple disciplines [SLP (Speech Language Pathologists), OT (Occupational Therapists), RD (Registered Dietitians), Psych (Psychologists), MD (Physicians), Nurse and of course parent] to define and name paediatric feeding disorders. The authors completed a manuscript which is currently in press (Goday et al. 2018). The next step to achieving Shannon's vision is to advocate for an ICD code specific to paediatric feeding disorder.

While the consensus paper and the ICD code will help with advocacy efforts for families that have children with paediatric feeding disorders, it was important for the organisation

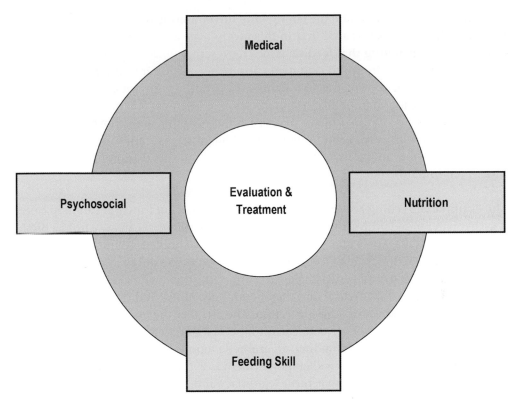

Figure 8.1 The different aspects in treating Paediatric Feeding Disorders
Reprinted with permission from Feeding Matters (https://www.feedingmatters.org).

to put this new definition in the ICF framework based on advice from their healthcare professional expert advisors. This advocacy organization partnered with professionals from several disciplines. The ICF served to situate the complexity observed by advocates and clinicians (see Fig. 8.1) of functional limitations into one framework that could describe the needs of that patient group in a consistent and standardized way.

The biological (biomedical) aspects of feeding disorders comprise what we find under the ICF's section on Body Functions and Structures, and many of them are defined by diagnoses affecting those functions and structures. Growth and Nutrition encompasses both body functions and also environmental factors. Skill & Ability describes Activities & Participation and Family, while Behavioural is a combination of environmental factors, activities and participation. This allows parents to have a broader understanding about how to address feeding problems. In becoming aware of all the factors involved, they can look for solutions (points of entry) beyond those usually associated with specific diagnoses found in the medical field. They value the input of different disciplines and the importance of having a shared view among all people involved in the evaluation and treatment of the child and the family. One survey among healthcare professionals from Feeding Matters revealed that in this group over 200 distinct diagnoses were represented, illustrating that feeding issues represent a *function* challenge (and not a 'condition' that 'belongs' to one medical subspecialty). Similar results could be expected if we were to bring together families of children with, for example, sleeping problems, restrictions in mobility, communication or interpersonal interactions – all of which are examples of impairments of people's *functions* that are almost never limited to, or treated exclusively within, one medical 'diagnosis' as traditionally conceived. Furthermore, there are rarely, if ever,disease-specific interventions for these kinds of functional impairments.

The example of Feeding Matters illustrates how the focus on function can help bring together parents and professionals around functional issues that can arise from a broad array of medical diagnoses and advocate together as stakeholders around one common goal. Starting from the issue of feeding, this group was successful in joining families of children with hundreds of varied diagnoses, connecting them with a network of distinct professionals of varied medical and therapeutic specialties, and driving the research with this approach towards a new direction. The fact that the group is advocating for the creation of a new descriptive diagnostic label is a sign that in the current environment of research and service funding, an umbrella term is still required. Perhaps their imaginative approaches so far will empower them to avoid falling back into the trap of needing a diagnosis in order to achieve legitimacy and perpetuating a 'class system of care' (Kraus de Camargo 2017)!

Policy applications

In Spain, a national survey on disability was established in 1986. The analysis of a sample from this survey using the ICF showed that many functional aspects of people's daily lives such as mobility and activities of daily living are well represented but that other aspects, especially those related to participation, are not identified and would require an adaptation of the survey tools to better describe the broader picture of the functional health of the population (Maierhofer et al. 2011).

References

Cibis W (2009) [The term 'Funktionale Gesundheit' (functional health) in the German edition of the ICF]. *Gesundheitswesen* **71**(7): 429–432.

Darrah J, Wiart L, Magill-Evans J, Ray L, Andersen J (2012) Are family-centred principles, functional goal setting and transition planning evident in therapy services for children with cerebral palsy? *Child Care Health Dev* **38**(1): 41–47.

Deutsche Interdisziplinäre Arbeitsgruppe zur ICF Adaptation für den Kinder- und Jugendbereich (2012) ICF-CY Checklists [online]. http://www.bvkm.de/servicematerialien/icf-checklisten-kinder-und-jugendliche-fuer-die-praxis-aufbereitet.html.

Deutsches Institut für Jugendhilfe und Familienrecht (DIJuF) e. V. (2015). *Datenschutz Bei Frühen Hilfen Praxiswissen Kompakt*. [*Data protection in early support systems*] edited by S. Nothhafft. Nationales Zentrum Frühe Hilfen (NZFH). https://www.fruehehilfen.de/no_cache/serviceangebote-des-nzfh/materialien/publikationen/einzelansicht-publikationen/titel/datenschutz-bei-fruehen-hilfen/

Goday P, Huh SY, Silverman A, Lukens CT, Dodrill P, Cohen SS, et al. (2018) Pediatric feeding disorder – Consensus definition and conceptual framework (in press). *J Pediatr Gastroenterol Nutr.*

Grotkamp S, Cibis W, Behrens J, et al. (2010) Personbezogene Faktoren der ICF – Entwurf der AG 'ICF' des Fachbereichs II der Deutschen Gesellschaft für Sozialmedizin und Prävention [Personal contextual factors of the ICF draft from the Working Group 'ICF' of Specialty Group II of the German Society for Social Medicine and Prevention]. *Gesundheitswesen* **72**(12): 908–916.

Kertoy MK, Russell DJ, Rosenbaum P, et al. (2013) Development of an outcome measurement system for service planning for children and youth with special needs. *Child Care Health Dev* **39**(5): 750–759.

Kraus de Camargo O (2007) Die ICF-CY als Checkliste und Dokumentationsraster in der Praxis der Frühförderung. *Frühförderung Interdisziplinär* **26**: 158–166.

Kraus de Camargo O (2017) Divide and Conquer – A Class System of Care [online]. https://medium.com/@DevPeds/divide-and-conquer-a-class-system-of-care-29dfc45ee106.

Kraus de Camargo O, Fayed N (2013) 'Health status' and the usefulness of the ICF framework: Clinical and Program perspectives. In: Ronen GM, Rosenbaum PL (eds.) *Health Participation and Quality of Life in Young People with Neurodevelopmental Conditions: Theory Concepts Evidence and Practice*. London: Mac Keith Press, pp. 36–50.

Leonardi M, Sykes C, Madden RCRH, et al. (2015) Do we really need to open a classification box on personal factors in ICF? *Disabil Rehabil* **38**(13): 1327–1328.

Maierhofer S, Almazan-Isla J, Alcalde-Cabero E de Pedro-Cuesta J (2011) Prevalence and features of ICF-disability in Spain as captured by the 2008 National Disability Survey. *BMC Pub Health* **11**: 897.

McDowell M, O'Keeffe M (2012) Public services for children with special needs: discrimination by diagnosis? *J Paediatr Child Health* **48**(1): 2–5.

Simeonsson RJ, Lollar D, Bjorck-Akesson E, et al. (2014) ICF and ICF-CY lessons learned: Pandora's box of personal factors. *Disabil Rehabil* **36**(25): 2187–2194.

Tantilipikorn P, Watter P, Prasertsukdee S (2012) Identifying assessment measures and interventions reported for Thai children with cerebral palsy using the ICF-CY framework. *Disabil Rehab* **34**(14): 1178–1185.

Vardiman JW, Harris NL, Brunning RD (2002) The World Health Organization (WHO) classification of the myeloid neoplasms. *Blood* **100**(7): 2292–2302. https://doi.org/10.1182/blood-2002-04-1199.

WHO (World Health Organization) (2007) *International Classification of Functioning Disability and Health – Children and Youth Version, 1st edn*. Geneva: World Health Organization.

Section C

Chapter 9

The ICF from the parent perspective

Jennifer Johannesen

My experience as a parent to a child with multiple severe disabilities lasted just a few short years; my son Owen died in 2010, at the age of 12. His early death was both surprising and wholly predictable – while he was in the midst of a particularly healthy spell, we had always known his life-long physical and developmental challenges would likely mean a shorter-than-average life. As Owen's full-time caregiver, I knew the amount of work required to simply keep him alive, never mind *also* trying to provide a good quality of life for him,as well as his younger brother, Angus (who is typically developing). I felt immensely grateful to the Canadian healthcare system as well as to our team of skilled and compassionate health professionals. At the same time, particularly as my experience and confidence grew, I became increasingly attuned to absurdities, redundancies, and confusing narratives that lived alongside the good care and technical excellence. Since Owen's death, I have been attempting to make sense of these contradictions by reflecting on our experiences and imagining new ways forward – including, as outlined in this book, considering use of the ICF in clinical practice.

Owen had what I think of as 'conventional' medical treatment – we were primarily focused on his physical health and considered his functioning in terms of 'normal' stages of development. Indeed, we had the good fortune to be treated by clinicians who were also caring, inquisitive and observant. Their biomedical approach was tempered by their maturity and experience, and, dare I say, by their humanity. It was their diagnostic and technical capabilities *combined with* their creative and sensitive approaches to figuring out how to help our family that made for enriching and successful interventions.

We also experienced the opposite end of the clinical encounter spectrum. My son's various diagnoses included profound hearing loss, spastic quadriplegic cerebral palsy, and dystonia. He was also non-ambulatory and G-tube fed. His requirement for supportive equipment and devices seemed endless, which meant we encountered many specialists whose skills were closer to those of engineers than physicians. For these types of specialists, our lives and contexts mattered only so far as they related to the use of a particular apparatus or that would be impacted directly by a particular intervention. There was little inquiry into the many minor and major intersections of Owen's or our family's life activities and experiences that may have been tangentially impacted.

Regardless of the type of encounter we experienced, there was little interprofessional communication. I was the conduit through which details of Owen's health and development were reported to others. Because I couldn't possibly know exactly which details would be important to which health professionals, I am quite sure my ability to relay pertinent and accurate information was less than perfect.

Reflecting on the biomedical paradigm

I learned about the ICF long after my son's death, but immediately saw how it might have improved some of our healthcare experiences. It offers a much-needed paradigm shift in terms of how clinicians see our disabled children, by including individual and family context, priorities, and goals as part of the health record. In addition, when the ICF concepts are well used, members of the healthcare team collaborate, aligning their care towards shared goals. I can imagine that use of the ICF in clinical practice will help healthcare teams better understand the perspectives of the individual and family.

Parents may also come to see their own situation and experiences in a different light. Parents may learn that adherence to a rigid trajectory of 'normal' development may impede discovery of opportunities for connection, fun, and access to social and public spaces. For example, a focus on developing walking as the sole means for a child to get around may delay or indeed impede the use of a wheelchair, which can provide independence and access to activities.

We had an experience that illustrates this. As a 2-year-old, Owen was still very much functioning as an infant – he was fully physically dependent and had little functional movement. I had saved up a pressing question for several months and finally worked up the nerve to ask Owen's neurologist, 'Will he ever walk?' The neurologist seemed to have anticipated the question. 'Well,' she said, 'typical child development follows a certain path. First, a child might lift his head, then look around, then decide he wants to get something and so figures out how to crawl. And so on.' I understood where she was going, even as my heart sunk – Owen hadn't yet even lifted his head. She continued to explain that we should look for developmental achievements in sequence so we don't get ahead of ourselves. I remember thinking it was a kind way to say no. I left our meeting with a renewed focus to work on head control.

When Owen died at the age of 12, he still couldn't hold up his head despite the many years of therapy. At some point I had indeed moved on and stopped focusing so much on this one particular 'skill', and with the help of his occupational therapists, trialled many different pieces of equipment to support sitting, standing, and walking. In his various therapies, there were several times he was clearly 'walking' (albeit with full body support), and although for Owen these efforts did not amount to functional ambulation, I was proud nonetheless. Upon reflection, I can see that our neurologist's well-intentioned explanation may have set me down a path that held me back from exploring other ways of 'walking' using assistive devices.

I don't know if our neurologist was aware of the ICF. She was certainly kind and patient, and interested in our lives and experiences. Perhaps more than anyone she understood that we would always be assessing Owen outside the boundaries of typical development. Yet, her academic training, combined with old habits, ran deep – I suspect the impulse towards biomedical framing was very strong. In many cases, perhaps even in this case, a biomedical view may be appropriate. However, if there had been an explicit effort to bring together our specialists to help address my own questions and priorities, I may have received a different or more comprehensive answer to my question about walking, thus helping me imagine a different future. The ICF, with its emphasis on individual and family priorities and goals, combined with its encour-agement for interprofessional dialogue and information sharing, makes it a robust patient-centric approach that can possibly offer fresh and productive directions for individuals and families.

Considering disability

Through the ICF lens, disability is considered not as a series of deficits within the per-son, but as a contemplation of the 'fit' between a person and their environment. When assessing an individual's needs from this perspective, we might more readily identify physical barriers that can be removed or adjusted, or better prepare social groups to include someone with particular communication needs. In other words, barriers and hindrances to accessing certain experiences can be located not exclusively in a person's diagnosis or physical limitation, but also in how we set up and maintain an environ-ment to support that person with their specific constellation of characteristics. The ICF framework allows a healthcare team, including the individual and family, to examine how a person lives and interacts with their environment, which can give important clues as to what interventions can be helpful. This strikes me as a respectful and person-centred approach to supporting an individual's needs and goals – more so than simply diagnosing a 'problem' and trying to fix it with a medical intervention.

This idea of determining fit is, of course, something that all people contemplate, not only those with disabilities. One could say that *all* people in a community live on a spectrum of needs, wants, and priorities. Therefore, everyone has needs and everyone requires some kind of intervention or accommodation; this reframing of disability challenges our assumptions and biases about what constitutes *normal*, which can create opportunities for a constructive shift for individuals and families.

While positive messaging and attitudes may be helpful, parents and professionals alike should consider that euphemisms can be confusing and misleading and can run counter to how some individuals feel about their identities. For example, some disability advocates reject the term 'differently abled', as it potentially erases their disability identity, and still carries stigma as it is not a term commonly applied to everyone (ADA National Network 2015, Dunn & Andrews 2015). Indeed, use of the ICF does not mean we no longer discuss symptoms and diagnoses. In fact, traditional labels can be helpful as long as they are accurate and descriptive, and accompanied by contextual and function-based information as described in the ICF.

When considering language choice and how a child's conditions and experiences are described, parents may wish to consider connecting with parents of older children and young adults, as well as adults with similar disabilities, to help broaden their own perspectives.

Decision-making

By the time Owen was 8 years old, I felt immensely overwhelmed with the types of decisions I was increasingly being asked to make. His 'interior' health, as I called it, was relatively stable. This meant his respiratory, circulatory, and digestive health all seemed to be functioning as expected. His spasticity and dystonia, on the other hand, were continuing to pose new and difficult challenges. I was concerned about his caregivers' ability (including my own) to continue to care for him safely, given his unpredictable movements and growing size. He had reached the tolerance thresholds associated with his oral medications, so our only recourse was to consider more invasive approaches that would potentially address his symptoms more directly. He had already had one implanted device, an intrathecal baclofen pump, which was eventually removed due to malfunction. We were now being asked to consider an invasive surgery that involved another implant – deep brain stimulation.

I felt overwhelmed because I became increasingly uncertain about how I ought to go about making decisions. I was concerned especially with the responsibility of making irreversible medical decisions on behalf of someone else, whose own wishes and priorities I might never know. I felt this acutely even though Owen was my own son. As well, trying to distinguish between his needs and my own was especially difficult, given how intertwined our lives were. Our health professionals were sympathetic and of course informative – I never doubted their advice and guidance from a biomedical perspective. However, when it came to this level of nuanced and deeply personal contemplation, it seemed to fall outside the scope of what they were able or felt willing to provide. Eventually I consulted a bioethicist in our local children's rehabilitation hospital, after which I concluded that even though I may make imperfect decisions, the responsibility to do so was indeed, appropriately, mine.

I share this story to illustrate the complexities and challenges some parents experience when making decisions, especially those that are emotionally fraught. Use of the ICF may create both opportunities and challenges for health professionals to support individuals and families while making difficult decisions, as well as navigating inner or interpersonal conflict. Certainly, having pre-established priorities and goals may help with assessing factors in ways that contemplating purely biomedical factors do not. For example, a surgical intervention may indeed increase range of motion for a child's hip, but the length of recovery time may compromise their ability to participate in a 'priority' activity, such as summer camp. Therefore, with this in mind, the family may choose a less invasive therapy, or may choose to delay surgery until after the preferred activity is completed.

In this simple story, we can see how a fuller consideration of biopsychosocial factors may help the individual and family arrive at an agreeable decision. However, in this example, there may be other concerns that are not accounted for in the ICF model. For example, the parents may disagree on whether an intervention is needed at all; or, the child may be fearful and insistent that he or she doesn't want any more surgeries.

These are complex issues that use of the ICF is not meant to address. However, given that use of the ICF may invite discussion about much more than physical health, it may reveal areas where consensus is difficult to achieve or where tensions already exist, whether between family members or among other members of the healthcare team. Because of this, use of the ICF in clinical practice should be undertaken as a means to *support* meaningful and robust dialogue, not *replace* it.

Does the ICF fit all families?

Owen was deaf and nonverbal, non-ambulatory, G-tube fed, highly spastic and dystonic, and had no clear language-based communication system. He could not indicate his preferences, let alone act on them. He could indeed express approval or disapproval through vocalisation, crying and laughing, and facial expression. He also could communicate pain and pleasure through those same means, as well as physical reaction. To some extent, those who knew him well could discern some of his preferences , some of the time. Regardless, Owen had no ability to place himself in or remove himself from situations. He could not make requests, nor could he communicate decisions. All Owen's activities, situations, locations, and positions were not only determined by me, but also *performed* by me (or a designated caregiver). Unless an experience was (1) passive (e.g. he was sitting or lying down), and (2) tactile (e.g. feeling the wind on his face or water on his hands) or visual (e.g. watching a movie or seeing birds flying overhead), Owen required a facilitator to literally move him to and through an activity. Whether intentional or not, he was often cued as to what an appropriate reaction looks like – he would mimic his facilitator's facial expression, then be assumed to be feeling the associated emotions. Given this, to what extent could we really discern Owen's own goals and priorities, which are key components in using the ICF?

Through the ICF lens, one might place a parental relationship in the realm of 'environmental factors'. In Owen's case, this seems insufficient – even absurd. It would be very difficult to separate where he ended, and I began. Certainly, his physical body was his own as were his bodily functions (e.g. swallowing, elimination, perspiration) – I did not control these aspects. However, his baseline physical health and functioning could only be maintained by my constant intervention. For example, because Owen couldn't reposition himself voluntarily, I would arrange his arms and legs for what seemed to be more comfortable positioning. I would decide each night which side he was going to sleep on. As well, I decided which direction he should face and how long he would hold certain positions. Almost every aspect of his experience of simply *being* was dictated by my decisions and actions.

So, in this context, what should we make of ideas such as 'participation' and 'functioning'? Although we didn't use the ICF as proposed in this book, we did have therapists and other health professionals who would describe and assess Owen using similar ideas and language. When I read through reports – even those to which I contributed or where my own words were recorded – I could see that none captured the reality of Owen's complete dependence or the degree to which I *manufactured*, in a sense, his experiences. For example, when I interpreted Owen's response to a thing as 'positive', we would simply do more of that thing. That thing, then, by virtue of repetition, became his 'favourite', and was documented as such. In short, I would string together a series of attributions until they formed a logical and satisfying narrative. This presents interesting problems, then, in terms of using the ICF as a means to help individuals and families report on subjective experiences such as 'participation' and 'functioning'. One challenge is that it may be difficult to determine whose goals and priorities are being recorded. A second challenge is that, despite best efforts, it may be difficult to determine who is actually doing the participating and functioning.

A third and possibly more concerning challenge arises when a category doesn't quite fit how the individual or family might describe their own experiences, and parents in particular may feel they have to come up with 'good answers' regardless. In our case, given the nature of Owen's severe disabilities, I would never have thought to describe Owen as 'participating' or 'functioning'. These would have been ideas suggested by a teacher or a therapist. When asked to describe Owen using similar categories (e.g. 'social skills'), I found creative ways to give an answer without outright lying. In fact, I would have felt I wasn't doing my job as his mother if I couldn't produce what I thought would be sufficient answers for each category presented.

This poses two interesting potential problems.

First, it highlights just how deeply all parties are socialised within the biomedical paradigm; not only the healthcare team members but also the individuals and families. Just as professionals are trained in accepted norms and practices, so too are parents. This is evidenced by my own need to develop a narrative according to what I thought was expected of Owen, as well as of myself as his parent. This means that, if it's the health professionals that 'use' the ICF with the individual and family merely answering questions or otherwise providing data for the professionals' use, it will be more difficult for people to see its relevance to individuals and families. Use of the ICF as described in this book will likely have more impact and will ultimately feel more satisfying for individuals and families if it is deployed for team collaboration, not patient interrogation. Ideally, individuals and families will take it up as a means to lead and manage their own interaction with the healthcare system. This does not mean that families are left on their own, nor does it mean they dictate the terms of their care. Rather, it means they feel empowered, for example, to take initiative, to explore creative ideas, to experiment within agreed boundaries, and to probe and question professional recommendations openly.

Of course, it may take time for all parties to feel comfortable with this shift from a biomedical paradigm, where the health professional traditionally dictates or leads interactions from a biomedical perspective. In the ICF approach, the focus is less about 'who is in charge' and more about what – and whose – needs, goals, and priorities take centre stage. These terms should be negotiated and continually reassessed by the whole care team, including the individual and family.

A second problem may arise when individuals and families inadvertently reorient their perspectives to fit the categories presented by the tool, as people may assume those categories are comprehensive and definitive. The risk is that the healthcare team may miss out on important clues and information that are integral to the person for whom they are providing care. To be clear, *any* tool is likely to present its own normative stance. In this case, using the ICF in clinical practice might discourage individuals and families from sharing their experiences through the lens of their own paradigm, which might not fit the stated ICF categories. This challenge may not easily be addressable, as underlying counter-narratives such as these do not tend to readily reveal themselves. As well, parties may have an interest in demonstrating or understanding a situation in a particular way – perhaps to preserve their role as 'expert', which may have been my own unconscious motivation as well. In addition, it may simply be asking too much of any healthcare team member to unpack and decipher such emotional and inner complexities. To some extent, it is reasonable, and respectful, to take at face value how an individual or family may choose to represent themselves. On the other hand, a healthcare team member – particularly one who is trusted by the family – may find opportunity to engage in an exploratory dialogue about such matters.

This issue applies not just to severe disability, but could also apply to situations experienced by people from other cultures, languages, and socio-economic realities, to name a few. On a popular blog hosted by Holland Bloorview Kids Rehab Hospital in Toronto, Jaqui Getfield describes moving to Canada from Jamaica with her twin boys, both of whom are diagnosed with Autism Spectrum Disorder (Getfield 2013). She compares Jamaican and Canadian parenting, noting that 'Jamaican mothers do not carry on incessant … chatter with children who themselves can't speak' and that it's unheard of for working mothers to conduct 'pretend play' sessions and arrange play dates. She notes, that, in Jamaica, adults 'are not expected to be integrally involved in unstructured free play'. These and other parenting differences made it difficult for her to adapt to the expectations of her son's health professionals. Of particular note is Ms. Getfield's observation about eye contact – in some communities, she says, eye contact from children is considered disrespectful and confrontational. Until she arrived in Canada she did not appreciate the 'cultural importance of eye contact as a means of communication' to Canadians. Her sons' lack of eye contact at two years old, therefore, was much less concerning to her than it seemed to be to the health professionals.

Ms. Getfield's experience highlights how easy it might be for healthcare teams to miss important cultural differences and interpretations if a tool deployed to support information-gathering does not allow for other ways of understanding a person's condition or situation. In this account, we might surmise that indeed her sons' lack of eye contact warranted further investigation – we should also, then, appreciate that normative expectations in Canada may be different than elsewhere. Individuals and families from immigrant, marginalised, or otherwise under-served communities may feel they need to adapt to the normative paradigm presented through a given tool, thereby pushing aside or suppressing their own perspectives.

Although use of the ICF in clinical practice is a more robust and dynamic way of capturing a person's life situation, it nonetheless asserts culturally normative ideas of how one ought to categorise and describe needs, priorities, and experiences. People are indeed free to accept, reject, or adapt its terms. However, if a health professional presents the framework to a family *even just as a point of discussion*, the act itself is suggestive of a 'right way' to think about things. As mentioned above,

I would not have thought of 'participation' as a way to describe Owen's activities. Yet, how could one introduce the language of ICF into our care without requiring me to orient my thinking towards 'participation' as a basis for evaluation? Even if I were to reject it as a relevant category for our family, my sense would be that we were deviating from a proposed 'standard'. The issue I raise here is that all frameworks, including the ICF, have a *point of view* and should not be mistaken for being neutral, even if highly flexible.

Of course, no tool could, on its own, tease out the nuanced and complex biases described in Ms. Getfield's account. As a result, as argued earlier here and elsewhere in this book, the tool should support, not replace, dialogue. Effective use of the ICF in clinical practice requires that clinicians be open to the ways that individuals and families in their care are conducting and experiencing their lives, even if the clinicians' own perceptions or impulses are different. This helps to safeguard against potential pressure a family may feel to conform to the perceived 'standards' of the tool, or indeed, the clinician. Categories presented in the ICF should serve as *prompts* for all parties to align around the needs and priorities of the people involved, which may require adapting or refining the tool itself, the associated consultative processes, or the perspectives of the healthcare team members, to more accurately reflect a family's life situation.

Back to basics

As described in the first two sections of this book, the ICF was not developed to be used in clinical practice to help individuals and families directly. It was first developed as a classification system by the World Health Organization, to more accurately reflect the functioning, needs and abilities of populations. For nations who might use the ICF at a federal policy level, it can help to determine current resource allocation requirements and also to anticipate future needs. But in order to do this effectively, the system needs data, which means it needs willing participants – clinicians and individuals alike – to use the associated instruments and contribute to ongoing data exchange activities. This framework needs to be implemented at ALL levels of healthcare, from international organisations, to federal health initiatives, to regional administrative bodies, all the way down to the clinic, and the home. A fully integrated system is required to support the two-way flow of communication that is vital to the entire analytical process. Individuals provide the data, the databases provide the statistics, the statistics (theoretically) inform funding decisions, which ultimately, should provide appropriate support and resources to communities and individuals.

It's all a rather grand vision which, in its entirety, might not be one that individuals and families have the time or energy to concern themselves with. Instead, individuals and families would need to determine for themselves that this framework supports or enhances the quality of their care, the nature of their family and care-provider relationships, and the ways in which they experience their activities and occupations. In other words, it needs to be meaningful to them in their everyday lives.

A common complaint among individuals and families is that their health professionals simply don't have enough time for them (Ogden et al. 2004). Modern healthcare, which is often under pressure to reduce costs, has failed to provide enough time and resources for health professionals to engage with their patients in a substantial way. At the same time the broader healthcare system, in Canada, is criticised for different reasons: it is perceived as administratively complex, and services are difficult to navigate (Grant 2017). For individuals and families, they may experience this in multiple ways. For example, they may feel there are too many specialists to keep track of, none of whom communicates with each other or has an overview of the 'big picture'. Families cannot provide or access centralised health records, and in fact must repeat their own story over and over again to different professionals. As well, they may feel their *experience* of their health is not well understood, despite all of the medical efforts to treat symptoms and conditions.

All of this, it seems, may be addressed by using the ICF in clinical practice. Individuals and families may feel their interests are more accurately captured in their health record. Health professionals may appreciate the collaboration and creativity of interprofessional dialogue. Subsequently, improvements in communication will hopefully lead to providing the most relevant and appropriate care for the individual, whether through medical interventions, environmental modifications, or supports of another kind. In one sense the ideas behind the use of the ICF seem novel. In another sense, they seem downright old-fashioned – perhaps the ICF approach represents a return to ideals of medicine that may have fallen away due to the biomedical institution's focus on efficiency and cost-savings.

Ways forward: Possible applications

The questions and considerations put forward in this chapter are complex and may not be resolved any time soon. These could best be thought of as ongoing queries that may come in and out of focus, as issues and opportunities arise through continued use and development of the ICF. I certainly do not suggest that considering these and other critical questions should delay or prevent clinicians, individuals, and families from working together to figure out how the ICF might support the individual and family.

The ICF approach does not necessarily need to be implemented as a permanent, exhaustive framework by which to assess everything, always. While none of these ideas has been tested or proven, I suggest a few ways one might consider integrating

ICF into clinical practice – either to 'test the waters' (potentially leading to a more robust implementation in the future) or as a selectively applied intervention at critical moments in the care journey of an individual and family. Although they are listed separately, one might imagine how use of the ICF can be beneficial in multiple ways.

- **As a dialogue tool.** The categories listed in the ICF could form the basis for either planned or spontaneous dialogue with an individual or family meant to stimulate creative problem solving, work through life-stage transitions, or otherwise encourage a fuller discussion of an individual's needs and priorities not elicited in routine clinical practice. As well, by focusing dialogue around common themes (such as 'environmental supports'), healthcare team and family members may find they are better able to articulate and align with shared goals, thereby reducing or avoiding conflict.

- **As a decision aid.** When considering the merits of a therapy, intervention, or major change in care routines, it may be helpful to use the ICF in discrete moments, to map out the expected as well as possible outcomes of a major decision and assess the potential impacts in terms that may be more relevant to the individual and family than would otherwise be explored in a conventional biomedical approach. For example, a family considering a range of augmentative communication devices for their young child may find it beneficial to consider not only the impact on language development, and also how the device will impact (for example) participation in a preferred sport.

- **As a planning and communications support tool for families.** The biomedical approach in clinical practice may feel safe and familiar for both families and healthcare team members. However, the ICF approach presents opportunities for individuals and families to *organise* their thinking towards needs, goals, and priorities, which may lead to improved communication between family members, enriched understanding of their own situation, and opportunity for reflection. Individuals and families may or may not choose to share resulting thoughts with healthcare team members. When used in this way, the tool is available to support families in whichever ways work for them.

- **As a compassionate intervention.** Individuals and families accept their diagnoses and associated characteristics to varying degrees; some integrate their conditions as an important part of their identity, while others, on the opposite end of the spectrum, deny their condition or hold out unreasonable hope for a cure. For most people, their reality exists somewhere in the middle. While pursuit of biomedical solutions may be productive and in fact entirely reasonable, it may also help individuals and families to experience progress in ways that do not rely on massive scientific breakthrough or innovation. By introducing non-biomedical considerations into the discussion, the ICF approach may bring a sense of possibility to a family at a time when biomedicine alone may provide little or none.

On a broader level, development and application of the ICF should continue in partnership with individuals and families. This should happen at policy levels as well as at community and interpersonal levels. Indeed, use of the ICF as a conceptual and communications tool in clinical practice should be negotiated with each individual and family – creative adaptations and variations may be required in order for everyone involved to feel its use is effective and practical.

References

ADA National Network (2015) *Guidelines for Writing About People With Disabilities*. https://adata. org/factsheet/ADANN-writing.

Dunn DS, Andrews EE (2015) Person-first and identity-first language: Developing psychologists' cultural competence using disability language. *Am Psychol* **70**: 255–264.

Getfield J (2013) Let's find the missing family-centred pieces. *BLOOM*, 16 December. http:// bloom-parentingkidswithdisabilities.blogspot.com/2013/12/lets-find-missing-family-centred-pieces.html.

Grant K (2017) Patients resort to paying consultants to help navigate Canada's Byzantine health-care system. *The Globe and Mail*, 14 April. https://www.theglobeandmail.com/news/national/ consultants-are-helping-the-sick-navigate-canadas-health-care-system/article34714551/.

Ogden J, Bavalia K, Bull M, et al. (2004) I want more time with my doctor: a quantitative study of time and the consultation. *Fam Pract* **21**: 479–483.

Chapter 10

Perspectives for future developments of the ICF: Challenges and suggested considerations

Olaf Kraus de Camargo

In comparison to other classification systems of the WHO (such as the International Classification of Diseases [ICD], now entering the 11th version in its more than 100 years of development), the ICF is still a very young classification system. The WHO website provides an update platform that can be used both for updating ICD codes and ICF codes. To contribute to further expansion of the ICF, as well as necessary corrections, interested users can register on the following website: https://extranet.who.int/icfrevision/ nr/loginICF.aspx and submit their suggestions. These are initially moderated online and then discussed during the annual meetings of the members of the Functioning and Disability Reference Group (FDRG) of the WHO Family of International Classifications (WHO-FIC). Initial developments of the ICF include the Children and Youth Version of the ICF in 2007; 10 years later most of the items that have been proposed for use with this young population have been integrated into the ICF, so that as of 2017 only one version of the ICF, covering the whole lifespan, will continue to be maintained by the WHO.

As expected for such a young classification, discussions are ongoing and focus on the framework, the content and the implementation of the ICF.

With regards to the framework, a group of researchers have proposed new depictions of the scheme for further discussion. The main aspect of these schemes is the integration of the box for 'Health condition' into the personal factors, based on the understanding

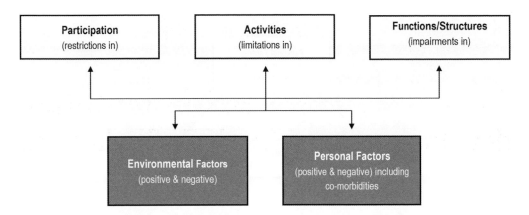

Figure 10.1 Alternative ICF Scheme 1
Heerkens et al. 2018. Reprinted with permission from Taylor and Francis.

that the whole framework describes health (Heerkens et al. 2018). Figures 10.1–10.3 provide examples of the proposed schemes.

Updating the ICF is a continuous process that includes adding necessary elements to the different domains, as well as possibly coming to a consensus for a list of personal factors (Leonardi et al. 2015, Heerkens et al. 2018), (though in our opinion these should not either be qualified or classified). The revision is an often challenging process that will lead to new versions of the ICF over time. The biggest challenge, though, continues to be the dissemination of this knowledge and the use of the ICF in clinical practice as

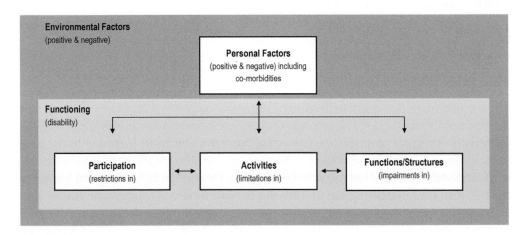

Figure 10.2 Alternative ICF Scheme 2
Heerkens et al. 2018. Reprinted with permission from Taylor and Francis.

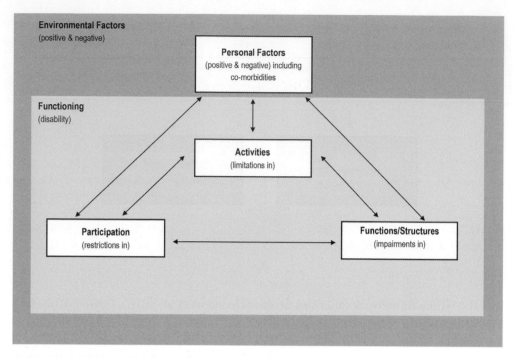

Figure 10.3 Alternative ICF Scheme 3
Heerkens et al. 2018. Reprinted with permission from Taylor and Francis.

well as a standard for evaluating population functional health. What are the challenges for further implementation?

• Lack of knowledge of the ICF.

• Variability of functional profiles.

• Lack of validity of qualifiers.

• Burden of documentation.

• The tradition of top-down collection of statistical data.

To become a regular part of clinical practice the ICF needs to be included in the core curriculum of all healthcare workers, educators and professionals in the areas of social work and welfare as well as the standard healthcare clinical fields. Beyond knowing the ICF and understanding the underlying biopsychosocial framework, it will also be important to convey the understanding that obtaining a functional profile of a person based on the ICF is very different from establishing a diagnosis (see Chapter 1). A functional profile must be understood in the context of a specific life situation, and it must be clear that these profiles can change over time. It is also important to understand that, depending on the observer's perspective, the focus of the functional profile can vary considerably according to the professionals involved and the topics that are raised during the encounter. Confronted with such variability, critics of the ICF easily mistake it as a lack of precision in comparison with established diagnostic criteria within the ICD. What is often not appreciated is that an individual's ICF profile is always a work-in-progress, a snapshot-in-time under a certain perspective, and hence liable to change as life circumstances change. This reality needs to be contrasted to the relative stability of 'diagnosis' based on biomedical dimensions of people's lives.

Another barrier for implementation is the uncertainty about how to use the qualifiers provided by the ICF. Theoretically the linear distribution of qualifiers according to the degree of impairment, limitation or restriction makes sense, whereas in practice it turns out to be quite subjective depending on the user of the ICF. For some items of the ICF there are established tools with good validity and reliability, and in those cases these results can be expressed using the distribution of the specific qualifiers. For example, different levels of 'functional mobility' in children with cerebral palsy can be well described using the reliable and valid Gross Motor Function Classification System (Palisano et al. 1997). For many areas, though, such tools do not yet exist, and the qualifiers become an arbitrary eye-of-the-beholder rating of the functional level with the descriptions of 'severity' using imprecise terms such as 'mild', 'moderate' and 'severe' to describe, for example, intellectual impairments. To allow greater acceptance and wider implementation of the ICF, it is probably helpful to avoid using qualifiers at all and rather identify areas of strength and weakness. Such a dichotomous description of a functional profile is sufficient to gather information that is relevant for the patient, allowing people to establish meaningful goals for intervention and to share these with all the professionals involved in the care. It also allows for the generation of significant functional information on a population level that goes beyond what exists based solely on diagnostic statistics that tell us nothing precise about functioning (see Chapter 8).

Every new type of documentation introduced into practice means an additional burden on staff. To facilitate implementation, the introduction of the ICF should make documentation work more efficient and less time-consuming. This requires a system that allows concomitant documentation by different team members as well as by the patients themselves. It must also allow the regular updating of functional profiles according to new life situations and changes in the health status and abilities of the patient.

Professionals will only adopt new tools and developments if they have been shown to benefit both the patient and the workflow of the professionals. One attempt to achieve both goals has been the development of 'Core sets' that are meant to reduce the number of ICF items and are designed to be specific to certain health conditions. In practice, these core sets still prove difficult to implement, as they remain quite lengthy; and since they have been developed for specific diagnoses, they frequently do not apply to the clinical reality of the multi-morbidity of patients with chronic health conditions and disabilities (McIntyre & Tempest 2007, Kraus de Camargo 2018).

For population statistics, there have been attempts to add ICF data to existing health statistics and to make their collection equally mandatory. Due to the additive character of producing a functional profile with the ICF the process of capturing relevant items/codes describing the situation of a patient can be quite variable depending on the situation, the professionals and family members involved, and the goals of the patient at a certain moment. Such a dynamic is very different from establishing diagnoses and coding them. This inherent variability of functional profiles requires that people communicate and re-evaluate such profiles on a regular basis. Delegating the selection of codes to coders, as is done with recording ICD codes in the healthcare system, might prove challenging and is frankly inappropriate.

For these reasons, a different approach to health statistics might be necessary. Instead of the top-down and mandatory pulling of data about patients from healthcare providers and organisations, data could be gathered bottom up, provided actively by citizens, patients and healthcare providers within a health information system. Such a paradigm shift is possible due to the ubiquitous availability of the internet and communication tools that allow sharing, collecting and analysis of data from all over the world. First attempts to develop such a platform are under way with the support of the WHO-FIC Functioning and Disability Reference Group and the establishment of an international collaborative for the **ICanFunction mHealth Solution** (*mICF*) (Snyman & Kraus de Camargo 2016):

> The vision for mICF is that this solution will empower **service users** (e.g. health, social, education) or their proxies to become 'agents' in their new role of 'directing' the process of service provision and care. They will be enabled to describe their own abilities in strengths and limitations (functioning) regarding the interaction with the existing environmental barriers and facilitators by using *mICF*. They will own their data; be free to securely share their information and consult with service providers; experience improved communication with their service providers to facilitate shared decision-making; exchange information anonymously with other users of *mICF* worldwide and therefore be better informed about their treatment and rehabilitation options (Snyman & Kraus de Camargo 2016).

Administrators will have anonymised data available for Big Data analysis. These data will contribute to improve global public health surveillance, which is the foundation for decision-making in public health. It will empower decision-makers to lead and manage more effectively by providing timely, useful evidence.

The Centers for Disease Control states in its CDC Vision for Public Health Surveillance in the 21st Century that 'with the increasing availability of clinical, insurer, social, and environmental data sets, the immediate challenge is to organize the data into a format that is accessible and useful for epidemiologists, statisticians, and others who might be able to use these data for public health surveillance. Until these data are available in a useable format, interpretation by subject matter experts is impossible and the data will not be useful' (Centers for Disease Control and Prevention 2012).

Another example of electronic developments using the ICF is the platform REHADAT ICF-GUIDE (https://www.rehadat-icf.de/en/) (German Economic Institute 2018). It is a website that, based on established linkings of ICF items, connects resources from the literature and also specific assistive devices from the Official Assistive Devices Catalogue in Germany to those ICF items. A person can use this guide to find specific literature or devices using ICF terms and domains as the searching structure.

Until powerful electronic systems are developed and available to make the ICF accessible for a broader population, other simplifications using pencil and paper have been suggested. In the Zurich Kanton in Switzerland, a standardised special education assessment using the ICF has been proposed. It contains a selection of ICF items that are anchored according to the main areas of special education support required for a child (Hollenweger 2015) (Table 10.1).

Another example is the Functioning Assessment Classification Tool (FACT) proposed as a means to organise relevant information for children requiring additional supports in school (Klein & Kraus de Camargo 2018) (see supplemental data: https://doi.org/10.3389/feduc.2018.00002). This tool describes two main aspects: (1) *functional* abilities along the areas of 'verbal', 'literacy', 'visual' 'executive', 'social' and 'self-regulation' abilities, and (2) *participation* restrictions at 'individual work', 'multistep task', 'group work', 'teacher directed group work', 'unstructured activity', 'structured physical activity' and 'unstructured physical activity'. Using this template, teachers, parents and clinicians can develop individualised education plans based on a consensus driven process.

Future applications of the ICF will probably integrate the existing paper and pencil solutions into electronic solutions that will have the added value of making it possible to develop functional profiles over a longer trajectory and also analyse aggregated data.

Those who feel that the ICF provides the right framework for the work they are doing with children and families are encouraged to see this as a starting point to 'compose' their own adaptations and tools that fit the needs of the people they care for and that are feasible within their working environment. The present book hopefully has provided stimulating ideas and examples from passionate advocates to change our focus from illness to wellness, from disability to function, and from exclusion to participation.

Table 10.1   The six indication areas for special education, their functional components and anchored items

Indication areas for special education and their functional components	Anchored ICF items
Cognition and Metacognition	
Cognitive functions	b164 – higher-level cognitive functions
Central functions for cognitive processing	b140 – attention functions
Functions closely related to cognition	d133 – acquiring language
Conscious sensory perception and sensations	
Seeing	b210 – seeing functions
Hearing	b230 – hearing functions
Pain	b280 – sensation of pain
Other conscious sensory perceptions	d120 – other purposeful sensing
Social-emotional functioning	
Emotions	b152 – emotional functions
Regulation of emotions, motivation and psychological energy	b130 – energy and drive functions
Social-emotional competencies	d720 – complex interpersonal interactions
Purposeful communication	
Operational aspects of communication	b310 – b330 voice and speech function and d330 – speaking
Motivational and social-emotional aspects of communication	d310 – communication with – receiving – spoken messages and d330 – speaking
Metacognitive aspects of communication	d330 – speaking and d335 – producing nonverbal messages
Movement, Mobility and motor functions	
Motor abilities	b735 – muscle tone functions and d410 – changing basic body position
Motor actions	b760 – control of voluntary movement functions and d440 – fine hand use
Execution of activities of daily living	
Single components are listed in the ICF	d230 – carrying out daily routine, d530 – toileting, d540 – dressing and d550 – eating

Translated and adapted with permission from Hollenweger 2015, p. 31.

References

Centers for Disease Control and Prevention (2012) CDC's vision for public health surveillance in the 21st century. *Morbid Mortal Weekly Rep* **61**(Suppl): 44.

German Economic Institute (2018) Rehadat ICF-Guide [online]. https://www.rehadat-icf.de/en/.

Heerkens YF, de Weerd M, Huber M, et al. (2018) Reconsideration of the scheme of the International Classification of Functioning disability and health: incentives from the Netherlands for a global debate. *Disabil Rehabil* **40**(5): 612–614.

Hollenweger J (2015) Indikationsbereiche – Ein Instrument des Kantons Zürich zur Klärung der Indikation für sonderschulische Massnahmen. *Schweizerische Zeitschrift für Heilpädagogik* **21**(2): 27–33.

Klein B, Kraus de Camargo O (2018) A proposed functional abilities classification tool (FACT) For Developmental Disorders Affecting Learning and Behaviour. *Front Educ* **3**: 2.

Kraus de Camargo O (2018) International Classification of Functioning Disability and Health Core Sets: moving forward. *Dev Med Child Neurol* **60**(9): 857–858.

Leonardi M, Sykes C, Madden RCRH, et al. (2015) Do we really need to open a classification box on personal factors in ICF? *Disabil Rehabil* **38**(13): 1327–1328.

McIntyre A, Tempest S (2007) Two steps forward one step back? A commentary on the disease-specific core sets of the International Classification of Functioning Disability and Health (ICF). *Disabil Rehabil* **29**(18): 1475–1479.

Palisano R, Rosenbaum P, Walter S, Russell D, Wood E, Galuppi B (1997) Development and reliability of a system to classify gross motor function in children with cerebral palsy. *Dev Med Child Neurol* **39**(4): 214–223.

Snyman S, Kraus de Camargo O (2016) mICF – ICanFunction MHealth Solution in the Making [online]. http://icfmobile.org/.

Appendices

Appendix 1   Case examples and exercises

Suggested exercise

By referring to the codes and their definitions from the complete ICF manual, or even from the reduced code sets available for download alongside this book (see Appendix 6), try to describe a child or patient you know well. You can also use one of the other examples from the book and look up the elements that you identified as relevant in the reports provided.

People doing this for the first time usually notice a preference for some components and items over others. They recognise those that are part of their day-to-day work as more familiar and easier to understand. To benefit from the breadth of the ICF it is recommended to look at all the components. You might discover how much additional information you know about the child even beyond the components of your initial preference. In doing so, you will also become aware of aspects that you do not yet know about the child or the child's environment. In this sense, the ICF is an invitation to gather more information, to aggregate it systematically, and to identify the connections among the elements of the framework. Even if you do not have that information, it allows you to identify who could provide the missing data and make appropriate interdisciplinary referrals accordingly.

Once you have achieved a complete description of the child, try to identify what – from your perspective and the perspectives of the family and the child – would be intervention goals. The following examples can illustrate how the information in the reports can be mapped to the ICF framework.

Case example: Carlos, male, 6 years old
Initial appointment

Carlos was born at term weighing 3.6 kg. He lives with his parents and an older sister, 10 years old, and a brother, 2 years old. As he grew he had always been smaller in size and below average on his growth curves.

In the past, Carlos had nonverbal communication in which he would gesture and point and communicate nonverbally. His mother reports that his language development was late.

Carlos has the support of a shared educational assistant (EA) who works predominantly with him. He prefers to play in isolation and rejects the advances of other children. When left to play by himself, he can be calm and content; however, whenever expectations are laid out, he becomes oppositional. He has a skin condition that will often cause extensive body rashes, itchiness and blotching. He is treated with an immunosuppressant, with limited success. Whenever Carlos has a flare, he becomes extremely irritable.

His mother reports that it is difficult to hold a conversation with him. He is always preoccupied by his own train of thoughts. The way he plays with figurines is mainly scripted from an action movie. He also presents with a fascination for numbers and time and measuring things. He is very inflexible in terms of moving to another idea and is mainly preoccupied with his own thoughts. He presents lots of repetitive and stereotyped behaviours.

He has multiple meltdowns at school and at home with difficulties with transitions. He likes certain routines for meals and daily activities. His mother notes that he must get dressed in a very particular way and gives him the same food in a specific way, otherwise he will not accept it. He can use utensils and feed himself; however, his mother helps him getting undressed. He can put his shoes on and take his socks off. He cannot do his zippers. It seems that Carlos can do many of these self-help activities independently; however, his mother takes over to get things done in time and avoid disruption. Carlos likes different kinds of toys, especially video games, blocks and Lego. He has an interest in building things and enjoys playing with toys. At school, he is agreeable with doing crafts; however, he refuses to present and show his work and emphasises this refusal by tearing his work apart after finishing. His mother has noted that he presents with scratching in difficult situations provoking anxiety.

Carlos goes to sleep at 8:00 p.m. with no difficulty falling asleep; however, he wakes up during the night periodically and plays with toys in his room. His mother does not know how many hours he will be up; however, he may have difficulty waking up in the morning, feels tired throughout the day and has naps, which sometimes happen at school. In terms of eating habits, Carlos has no dietary restrictions. He is not a picky eater. He likes orange food, however, in certain routines. His mother had described pica behaviours where he would eat dirt, snow and play dough. It seems that Carlos likes to explore the environment by sensory stimulation for exploration more than for dietary reasons. He also has trouble with excessive stimulation such as light or noise. He frequently complains that light hurts his eyes and dislikes hearing people singing or loud noises. He also does not like his head to be touched and does not allow his hair to be washed. His mother previously had described that Carlos used to have repetitive behaviours like spinning, banging his head and dragging his head on the floor as if he were vacuuming. These behaviours are not an issue now. In terms of language, his mother describes Carlos imitating and uttering words from TV shows extensively. He started stuttering about a year and a half ago. Whole and part word repetitions are reported as well as blocks during which Carlos stomps his foot, bangs his hand, turns his head, and his face turns red. At times, he will not engage in conversation appropriately and seems not to answer questions, or have tangential language display. He has a wide vocabulary and can speak 100% intelligibly. He has no difficulty in articulation apart from stuttering. He has adequate receptive speech.

Physical examination
Carlos's weight was 19.6 kg (50th percentile), height 105 cm (10th percentile). He was cooperative with examination, however, showed anxiety and asked several questions about needles and the details of the examination. He looked dysmorphic with depressed nasal bridge, undeveloped philtrum, and his head shape showed frontal bossing and dolichocephaly. His ears were of normal size and insertion. He had a high arched palate, with full cheeks and lips; his uvula was midline and teeth were normal. He had clinodactyly of 4th and 5th fingers bilaterally, with regular palmar creases. He had extensive patches of eczema on his face and extremities and trunk. Chest and abdomen examination were unremarkable. His gait showed some toe walking especially when running. He could put the heels down if prompted. There was good muscle tone and strength in all extremities. Carlos could rise from the floor with no difficulties, could hop on one foot for a long time, and was able to jump. Carlos was holding a crayon with an immature grasp but could print his name and recognise letters easily. He could draw a square and triangle and draw a person with details. He had good eye contact during the interaction. He seemed to enjoy praise significantly. Joint attention was preserved. He could wait for his turn and followed directions appropriately. He was sitting still in his chair and showed good focus. His repertoire of words was extensive; however, words for his developmental age were used based on repetitive speech from previously heard phrases and sentences, and his language was scripted. He was reluctant to follow new ideas and showed persistence in following his own agenda.

He had extensive dermatitis lesions on his ankles and wrists bilaterally, as well as involvement of his scalp and face. These lesions tended to bleed and ooze and there was abundant flaking. They tend to itch a lot, especially during episodes of anxiety.

Impression and plan

Carlos has Autism Spectrum Disorder. Currently, however, Carlos's atopic dermatitis is severely affecting his quality of life, as he is also missing school frequently and there is a lack of attention at school. Today we have filled out all the necessary forms have taken consent for IVIG (intravenous immunoglobulin) which will take about 2–3 weeks to initiate. In the meantime, he was prescribed prednisone for the skin lesions.

Diagnoses

• Autism spectrum disorder

• Severe atopic eczema

• Stuttering.

In collaboration with the family the following priority goals were identified:

1. Carlos will understand when he needs to use self-regulation strategies and be able to verbalise options.

2. Carlos will be able to tolerate hair washing with shampoo.

3. Using tools such as noise-cancelling ear phones or self-soothing techniques, Carlos will be able to tolerate environments with loud noises at home and in the community.

4. Carlos will be able to use a variety of self-soothing techniques in the morning, prior to going to school.

Below you will find an ICF-informed functional profile based on the descriptions in the report above. It allows us quickly to visualise the main issues and strengths as a basis for the discussion and shared decision-making about the goals to be achieved.

Functional Profile - Carlos

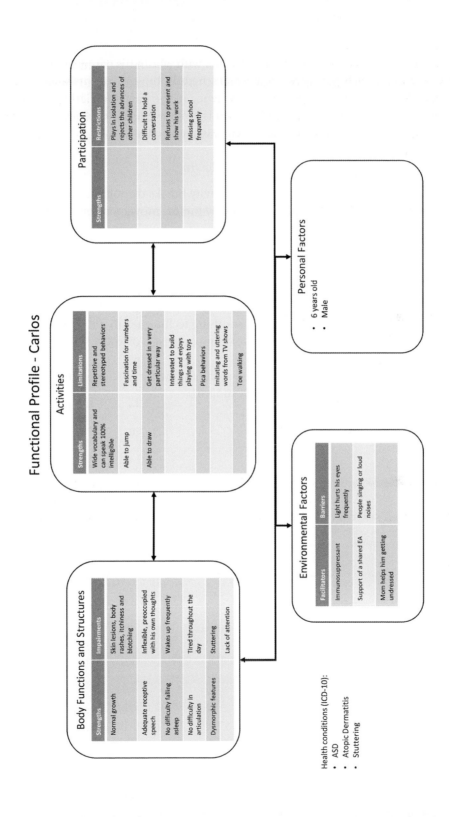

Body Functions and Structures

Strengths	Impairments
Normal growth	Skin lesions, body rashes, itchiness and blotching
Adequate receptive speech	Inflexible, preoccupied with his own thoughts
No difficulty falling asleep	Wakes up frequently
No difficulty in articulation	Tired throughout the day
Dysmorphic features	Stuttering
	Lack of attention

Activities

Strengths	Limitations
Wide vocabulary and can speak 100% intelligible	Repetitive and stereotyped behaviors
Able to jump	Fascination for numbers and time
Able to draw	Get dressed in a very particular way
	Interested to build things and enjoys playing with toys
	Pica behaviors
	Imitating and uttering words from TV shows
	Toe walking

Participation

Strengths	Restrictions
	Plays in isolation and rejects the advances of other children
	Difficult to hold a conversation
	Refuses to present and show his work
	Missing school frequently

Environmental Factors

Facilitators	Barriers
Immunosuppressant	Light hurts his eyes frequently
Support of a shared EA	People singing or loud noises
Mom helps him getting undressed	

Personal Factors

- 6 years old
- Male

Health conditions (ICD-10):

- ASD
- Atopic Dermatitis
- Stuttering

143

Follow-up appointment after 1 year

Carlos now attends Grade 2, has a male teacher with whom his parents report they have a very good relationship. Carlos has a visual schedule, but the parents suggested to not have an EA this year as there was no consistency in the past and Carlos was felt to be relying too much on the EA. Overall, school is going well. Carlos does read very well, and he receives 1:1 support from his teacher, when needed.

At follow-up Carlos' mother reported the following:

- Carlos is frequently receiving half-hour activity breaks throughout his day and his mother finds this very helpful. He especially prefers movement breaks. He also finds the breathing exercises useful.

- Hair washing routine has improved; again, the family is using the breathing technique.

- Recently, loud noises have not been an issue. The family is going to purchase noise-cancelling earphones for a future trip to an amusement park.

- His mother could list a variety of self-soothing techniques that they now have in their repertoire (movement breaks, breathing exercises, comfort blanket, hugs etc.).

The functional profile below can be used at the follow-up to identify the changes that have occurred and plan the next steps of support.

Functional Profile - Carlos (2)

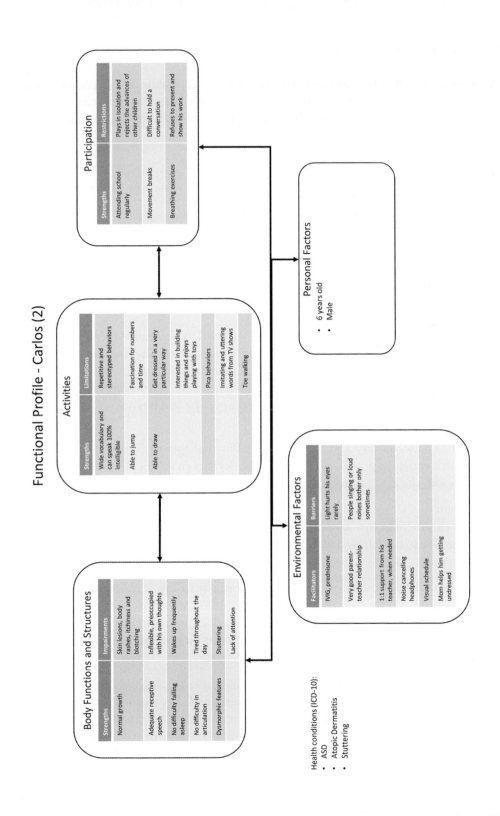

Body Functions and Structures

Strengths	Impairments
Normal growth	Skin lesions, body rashes, itchiness and blotching
Adequate receptive speech	Inflexible, preoccupied with his own thoughts
No difficulty falling asleep	Wakes up frequently
No difficulty in articulation	Tired throughout the day
Dysmorphic features	Stuttering
	Lack of attention

Activities

Strengths	Limitations
Wide vocabulary and can speak 100% intelligible	Repetitive and stereotyped behaviors
Able to jump	Fascination for numbers and time
Able to draw	Get dressed in a very particular way
	Interested in building things and enjoys playing with toys
	Pica behaviors
	Imitating and uttering words from TV shows
	Toe walking

Participation

Strengths	Restrictions
Attending school regularly	Plays in isolation and rejects the advances of other children
Movement breaks	Difficult to hold a conversation
Breathing exercises	Refuses to present and show his work

Environmental Factors

Facilitators	Barriers
IVIG, prednisone	Light hurts his eyes rarely
Very good parent-teacher relationship	People singing or loud noises bother only sometimes
1:1 support from his teacher, when needed	
Noise cancelling headphones	
Visual schedule	
Mom helps him getting undressed	

Personal Factors

- 6 years old
- Male

Health conditions (ICD-10):
- ASD
- Atopic Dermatitis
- Stuttering

145

Case Example: Jessica, female, 3 years 2 months
Diagnosis
Was born prematurely at 31 weeks (ICD 10: P07.3). Global developmental delay (ICD 10: F70.0) after septicaemia by meningococci and Waterhouse Friedrichsen syndrome (ICD 10: A39.1); Hydrocephalus with shunt (ICD 10: G91.2); Amputation of the left distal foot and right toes.

Interventions and therapies
Jessica has received early intervention in the last two years. She also receives physiotherapy 4–5 times per week.

Observations from Early Childhood intervention specialist
General impression
Jessica is a friendly and social girl. She reacts with joy when being addressed and new opportunities are offered to her.

Sensory
Jessica is initially reluctant and careful when exposed to new experiences. With a playful approach, she eventually takes new risks and enjoys them. She likes actions involving her body, especially when in contact with other people. She loves to swing and explores tactile stimulation with foam, play dough and finger paint. A hearing assessment was not feasible at the first attempt as Jessica did not comply. She also has not yet had a vision test.

Gross motor
Jessica can crawl quickly and with dexterity. She manages to climb up onto the couch and sit in a variety of positions. She has orthotics that enable her to walk while pushing a cart. Soon, she is to receive a walker.

Fine motor
The development in this area is delayed but Jessica is showing an increased interest in drawing. She tries to draw a face. She also enjoys cutting and string beads.

Cognition
It seems that Jessica's ability to learn varies from day to day. It can happen that on one day she knows all the colours and arranges objects by colour, but the next week she is unsure about this and a week later she again does not seem to have any difficulties identifying colours when dealing with finger paint. In general, her cognitive development does not seem age appropriate.

Language
Jessica's speech is unclear and difficult to understand. She cannot yet produce all the sounds. Her vocabulary is reduced. She has weak oral motor control and is unable to blow. On the other hand, Jessica likes to use her language to communicate and initiate social contact. She enjoys when others sing to her, preferably interacting with the whole body and making sounds accompanying the melody.

Play and social behaviour

Jessica has not had many opportunities to interact with children of her age. When she meets other children, she reacts with joy. When we went for a visit to a kindergarten she immediately wanted to stay there. She would benefit by participating in our integrative play group until being admitted at the kindergarten.

Her concentration and perseverance have improved but she still requires support to not give up easily when she encounters difficulties.

Recommendation

Due to her global developmental delay (see test results attached) and her physical limitations, Jessica has a high need for an 'integration spot' in kindergarten. This is to happen this summer.

The main functional aspects described in the report have been summarised, below, in the ICF framework. This overview provides a snapshot of her functional profile that can be shared and used as a reference to discuss points of entry for interventions and supports.

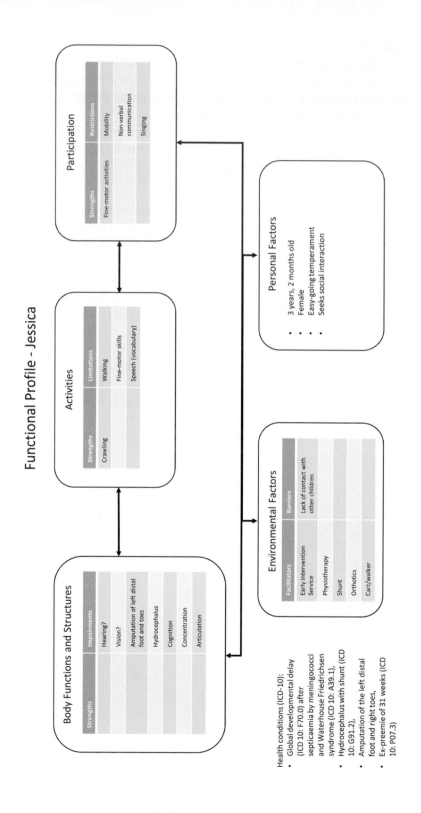

Functional Profile - Jessica

Participation

Strengths	Restrictions
Fine-motor activities	Mobility
	Non-verbal communication
	Singing

Activities

Strengths	Limitations
Crawling	Walking
	Fine-motor skills
	Speech (vocabulary)

Body Functions and Structures

Strengths	Impairments
	Hearing?
	Vision?
	Amputation of left distal foot and toes
	Hydrocephalus
	Cognition
	Concentration
	Articulation

Environmental Factors

Facilitators	Barriers
Early Intervention Service	Lack of contact with other children
Physiotherapy	
Shunt	
Orthotics	
Cart/walker	

Personal Factors

- 3 years, 2 months old
- Female
- Easy-going temperament
- Seeks social interaction

Health conditions (ICD-10):
- Global developmental delay (ICD 10: F70.0) after septicaemia by meningococci and Waterhouse Friedrichsen syndrome (ICD 10: A39.1),
- Hydrocephalus with shunt (ICD 10: G91.2),
- Amputation of the left distal foot and right toes,
- Ex-preemie of 31 weeks (ICD 10: P07.3)

Case Example: Paula, female, 5 years

Paula is her parents' only child. During the pregnancy, her parents lived in a refugee camp in Thailand where Paula was born. According to the parents the delivery occurred prematurely, and Paula's birth weight was 1 700g. On the second day of life Paula became quite jaundiced and had to be transferred to a hospital far away from the refugee camp. The parents were notified that her situation had deteriorated and that she would probably not survive. After 3 months, the parents received the news that her daughter had survived and that she would be transferred back to the refugee camp. They were informed that Paula required several blood transfusions and had to be ventilated.

During the first year of life Paula did cry a lot and struggled to drink from the bottle. She did not gain much weight. When she cried, her whole body became stiff and she arched her back.

Paula is 5 years old now and presents with the following medical diagnoses:

- Periventricular leukomalacia (ICD10: P91.6).

- Encephalopathy after kernicterus (ICD10: P57.0).

- Bilateral severe hearing loss (ICD10: H91.0).

- Vision impairment (ICD10: H53.9).

- Cerebral palsy GMFCS III with athetosis (ICD10: G80.4).

The family lives with the parents of Paula's father in a 2-room apartment on the second floor. The apartment itself has two levels and to reach the bedrooms it is necessary to take a flight of stairs. Both parents attend a language and integration course. During the home visit the father describes Paula's difficulties:

> She hardly can hear and recently has been fitted with hearing aids. At the beginning, she tried to pull them off, but her father managed to help her tolerate them better by putting in the hearing aids every time they would leave the house to go to the playground or do some grocery shopping. As Paula would require wearing a toque this helped to maintain the hearing aids in place and it was easier to distract Paula in the new environment, so she would not pull off her hearing aids. She does not have verbal communication and due to her motor difficulties is only able to point or direct her gaze vaguely into the direction of interest.

At home, she manages to get around by scooting on the floor. Frequently she tilts her head and seems to prefer a certain angle to look at objects. She loves a variety of toys. She can complete simple peg puzzles but requires a lot of determination to manage her eye-hand coordination. Paula likes to draw with crayons and produces lines and spirals.

With regards to her eating habits the father reports that the parents need to feed Paula and she only rarely has the patience to pick up food on her own and bring it towards her mouth. She drinks using a bottle or from a cup with a lid. She cannot dress or undress herself and depends completely on external help for this. During the nights, she sleeps well.

The grandparents have a limited understanding of Paula's disability. The parents feel emotionally very well supported by them but indicate that due to their advanced age they cannot support Paula physically.

Paula was prescribed a helmet due to her frequent falls. She also has a cart to be transported in the community, a special toilet seat and a special high chair.

Her father reports that Paula does not accept wearing the helmet. The toilet seat was prescribed to prepare Paula to use a toilet once she starts school. The parents report that Paula seems to feel very insecure when sitting on it and avoids being put on the toilet. The cart is used a lot when the family takes Paula out in the community. The high chair requires too much space and does not fit into the apartment. It is being used in kindergarten.

Assessment

During the developmental paediatric consult, Paula seems very restless and anxious when being undressed. The parents report that the many doctors' visits have led to fear from doctors and clinical investigations. Her movements present with dystonia and spasticity as soon as she initiates them. She tries to pull up herself to the standing position and raises her heels. After a while she relaxes and when held at the hips her heels slowly come down and touch the floor. To reach and grab objects her arm movements are uncoordinated and athetotic. She prefers to use her left hand. She is not able to follow an object with her eyes. The eyes present with an intermittent esotropia. It seems that the right eye is the leading eye. Her teeth are of yellowish-brown colouration, present with enamel hypoplasia and irregular surface. Paula does not allow herself to be examined or touched, starting to cry at the first attempts to do so.

Functional Profile - Paula

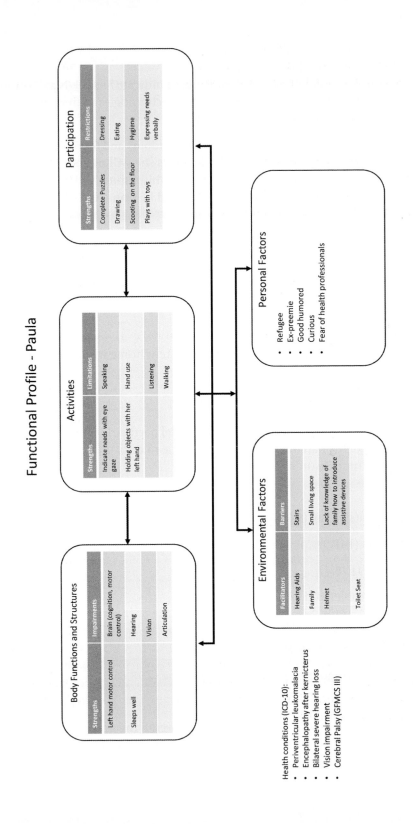

Body Functions and Structures

Strengths	Impairments
Left hand motor control	Brain (cognition, motor control)
Sleeps well	Hearing
	Vision
	Articulation

Activities

Strengths	Limitations
Indicate needs with eye gaze	Speaking
Holding objects with her left hand	Hand use
	Listening
	Walking

Participation

Strengths	Restrictions
Complete Puzzles	Dressing
Drawing	Eating
Scooting on the floor	Hygiene
Plays with toys	Expressing needs verbally

Environmental Factors

Facilitators	Barriers
Hearing Aids	Stairs
Family	Small living space
Helmet	Lack of knowledge of family how to introduce assistive devices
Toilet Seat	

Personal Factors

- Refugee
- Ex-preemie
- Good humored
- Curious
- Fear of health professionals

Health conditions (ICD-10):
- Periventricular leukomalacia
- Encephalopathy after kernicterus
- Bilateral severe hearing loss
- Vision impairment
- Cerebral Palsy (GFMCS III)

Intervention goals for Paula and her family

Using communication technology (d360)

Assistive technology might be helpful for Paula to indicate her needs and wants. It will be necessary to try out different approaches and technologies to find an adequate one for her that she is able to operate consistently.

Products and technology for mobility indoors and outdoors and for transportation (e1201)

This is a medium to long-term goal. As Paula grows she will not be able to use the cart anymore and will require a powered wheelchair. At this point it will be helpful to expose her and teach her how to use a joy-stick. This could be done in collaboration with the assistive technology support for communication.

Using a toilet (d530)

This is an important step for independence. The fear of sitting on the toilet is probably related to her lack of body control. It will be necessary to find ways together with the parents as to how to desensitise her and create an environment and supports that allow Paula to feel safe while sitting on a toilet.

Habitation services (e5250)

In the medium term the family will require a different home without stairs, more space and better accessibility.

Case Example: Peter, male, 6 years

Today we saw your patient Peter for a developmental paediatric consult. He came accompanied by both of his parents and was referred due to difficult behaviours and a query of Autism Spectrum Disorder (ASD).

Diagnoses

1. Developmental delay (R62.8).

2. Anxiousness (F41.9).

3. Stereotypies (F98.4).

4. Behaviour problems (F69).

5. Concomitant strabismus (H50.4).

6. Hearing loss in right ear (H91.9).

7. Status post myringotomy with insertion of tube (Z98.8).

History

Peter is the second of twins. According to his parents the pregnancy was uneventful and without complications. Delivery occurred about 1 month before the expected due date via C-section. Peter required some continuous positive airway pressure (CPAP) ventilation and tube feeding for about 5 days and was discharged at the age of about 10 days. He was bottle-fed until 1-year-old, and had no problem to transition to solid food. Regarding his milestones, the parents report that he was always a bit behind his twin sister and still is.

Developmental delays were first noticed when he entered day-care at age 18 months. At that time, he was not interacting with the other children, keeping mostly to himself and adults. Peter was seen here at our Centre by Occupational Therapy for fine motor and self-help issues and Behavioural Therapy due to aggressive behaviours when not getting his way. It was noted that he struggled in establishing social contacts with the other children at day-care and preferred to play on his own. He also was described having several sensory issues and sticking to routines and stereotypic play, getting upset when routines were disrupted. These observations resulted in the referral for today's consult.

Current concerns

Home

The parents report that in the home Peter does a lot of screaming, hitting and kicking mostly directed towards his mother, when he does not get his way. In one instance, he took a butter knife and pointed it at his sister. He continues to be fixated on certain routines and has meltdowns when they are broken. When asked or offered something he always rejects it or wants the opposite of what has been offered. He is also observed to be talking in a whispering voice to himself in a repetitive way. The parents observe that he looks up and to the right when he seems to be thinking through something. They report that he continues to be behind about 1 year in his fine motor skills and overall learning. They observe that he is afraid to fail and often gives a wrong answer although he knows the right answer, making a joke out of the situation.

He is observed to pat the floor and smell his hands and food before eating and 'strums' on his cheeks, palms of hands and feet. He tends also to have meltdowns when he is expected to wait and yells at his mother to listen to him 'now'. He always wants to anticipate what will be happening next and checks it over and over. He more recently is also displaying additional self-stimulating sexualised behaviour.

School

Peter is tired all the time. He is about 1 year behind academically, he does not yet know the colour yellow and does not know the letters a, q, d, p, l, b, h, P, D, Z, V. At school his behaviour is also defiant; all the doors need to be closed and he seems to be attracted by water, observing it flowing over his hand. He is a flight risk and has already wandered out of the classroom, having to be brought back by another teacher. He often seems to be in his own world, lying on the carpet for most of the day watching the wheels of cars and trucks. He has frequent injuries due to bumping into things and not watching where he is going (possibly also due to a vision problem). When instructions are given to the class, he remains on the floor without understanding what he is supposed to do. The teacher is worried about the transition to Grade 1 as at this point he is requiring 1:1 support from the Early Childhood Educator (ECE).

Health review

Peter is being followed by Ear, Nose and Throat Specialist (ENT) and has tubes in both ears as well as a hearing loss on the right side which will be addressed by a unilateral hearing aid. He will also be seen by Ophthalmology to receive a surgical correction of his strabismus. According to his parents in the past he did not see very well and was considered 'clinically blind'. This has improved.

No other health concerns.

Sleep

Talks in his sleep, sleeps through most of the nights.

Strengths

Peter has a great interest in the ukulele and is having lessons with some good progress. His music teacher adapts to him and follows his lead, doing what Peter enjoys.

Family composition

Cathy: twin sister, is in the same classroom, no problems at school and at home. Usually takes the lead and 'mothers' Peter when they play together. Peter seems quite attached to her.

Dad: has anxiety, on medication, well managed.

Mother: had some academic difficulties as a child, feels that she did not have the necessary attention, also has anxiety, on medication, grieving the loss of her father in December, works as an Educational Assistant (EA).

Pets: The family has a dog.

Observation and vitals

Peter came to the exam room and greeted me when prompted. After we said his name he corrected me how to pronounce it correctly. He made eye contact, smiled and tried to make fun. Initially, he did not want to play with any of the available toys, and after a while he got bored and said he wanted to leave. While standing at the door he would measure his parents with his eyes to anticipate their reaction. Once we blocked the door he lay on the floor and started whining but was distractible by his mother who picked some cars for him to play with. He did not engage in interactive play but rather would move the cars back and forth on the floor but maintained a conversation with his mother about their dog being upset at home. Towards the end of the consult, he was allowed to watch videos on a cell phone. He found the video of his teacher playing ukulele and showed it to me sharing that the teacher was behaving silly and laughing at this. No mannerisms or sensory issues were observed. Height: 112 cm (25th %ile), Weight: 18 kg (18th %ile).

Impression and plan

Peter is a 5-year-old boy with some health and developmental challenges that at this point cannot be attributed to one single diagnosis. On one hand, he presents with several features found in children with ASD, like being fixated on routines, stereotypic play and sensory issues. On the other hand, he seems to be quite capable of communication at his developmental level, interjecting, asking questions, arguing and sharing his enjoyment as well as anticipating emotions and actions of the people around him. One major contributor to his challenging behaviours could be a certain propensity to anxiety characterised by his fear of failing, his need to anticipate future events and his need for order. It could be hypothesised that his early vision and hearing difficulties associated with overall developmental delays led him to rely more on other senses like touch and smell as well as requiring a predictable environment around him.

We explained to the parents that due to Peter's complex presentation we do not feel that at this point we can come up with a diagnosis like ASD but that he certainly will require intensive support also in Grade 1. It will be important for him to create opportunities for the development of a trusting relationship with a teacher and EA in order to start engaging in learning situations more consistently. It might be helpful to have the behavioural team from the schoolboard involved in this as well. For the home situation, we re-referred the parents to our behavioural therapist and we had a short discussion about establishing logical consequences for certain behaviours and the importance of consistency to avoid mixed messages to Peter. A follow-up was offered in about 6 months to re-evaluate the situation.

Analysis

The reason for referral was a query for Autism Spectrum Disorder. In some school systems, this is an important question to clarify as it allows access to services for the student. Not making the diagnosis carries the risk that the child will not receive supports in the amount available for a child with similar needs but with that diagnostic label. Establishing a functional profile can help to elucidate the areas where help is needed, independent of the diagnosis and allow services to be implemented even before it is possible to establish a diagnosis with more certainty.

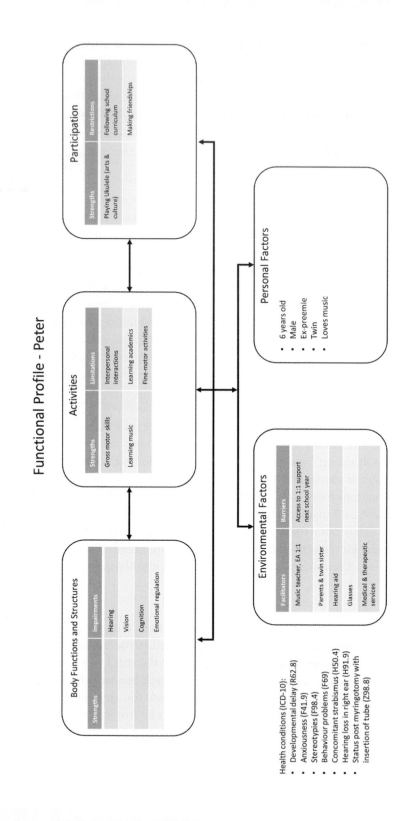

Functional Profile - Peter

Participation

Strengths	Restrictions
Playing Ukulele (arts & culture)	Following school curriculum
	Making friendships

Activities

Strengths	Limitations
Gross motor skills	Interpersonal interactions
Learning music	Learning academics
	Fine-motor activities

Body Functions and Structures

Strengths	Impairments
	Hearing
	Vision
	Cognition
	Emotional regulation

Environmental Factors

Facilitators	Barriers
Music teacher, EA 1:1	Access to 1:1 support next school year
Parents & twin sister	
Hearing aid	
Glasses	
Medical & therapeutic services	

Personal Factors

- 6 years old
- Male
- Ex-preemie
- Twin
- Loves music

Health conditions (ICD-10):
- Developmental delay (R62.8)
- Anxiousness (F41.9)
- Stereotypies (F98.4)
- Behaviour problems (F69)
- Concomitant strabismus (H50.4)
- Hearing loss in right ear (H91.9)
- Status post myringotomy with insertion of tube (Z98.8)

Appendix 2 Team development phases

Table 1 Team development phases

The Basic Group	This is the starting point for healthy team development.

As the group forms, the concern of each group member is that of **alignment:** that is whether they and other group members are all going in the same direction. There is a series of questions that each member is asking themselves as they join a new group. These questions are often asked sub-consciously, and are: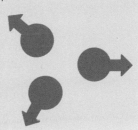

- 'Is this group going where I want to go?'

- 'Do I want to go where this group might be going?'

- 'Is being part of this group in my best interest?'

- 'Do I really want to be a part of this group?'

If each member doesn't get good answers to these questions, the **willingness** of some in the group to cooperate will be quite low.

As the group is newly formed, the inexperience of the group in working together will also have an impact on the level of **skill** in cooperation, which is likely to be low at the outset. Although individual members of the group may be quite skilled in certain team processes, it is the overall skill of the group that is important here.

In a group, things are done in a somewhat mechanistic, by-the-book manner. Feelings and true opinions are not expressed openly, because there are too many unknowns. Members are wary of each other. There is not much trust being shown. People are sizing each other up!

In the Basic Group, the focus of the members is on their own self-interests. In diagrams of the Basic Group you will often see arrows pointing in different directions. Until team members can answer the question of whether they want to be a part of the group, there is little chance that they will get to the next stage of team development. In fact, many groups never get beyond this first stage of development.

If there is good leadership and a clear task, the team will often appear to be effective – and to a limited extent, they are. However, results are more likely to be additive rather than synergistic. The power of this group lies in its potential rather than its current performance.

Summing up: the core issue of this stage is Alignment: do I want to go where the other members of this group want to go?

(Continued)

Table 1   (Continued)

The Adolescent Team	If and when team members become somewhat convinced that being a member of this group is in their best interest, they begin to move into the second stage of development – the Adolescent Team. 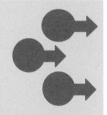
	They have now moved up the **willingness** scale, but still need to develop cooperation **skill** together.
	In this stage, the Team members become willing to risk being more open, and more willing to express personal concerns and feelings. Their attention begins to turn from personal to interpersonal concerns.
	Trust is the core issue at this stage. The focus of the team members is on getting to know their co-workers – their strengths, weaknesses and the unique contributions each brings to the team. Through this knowledge and the process of sharing it, trust begins to build, and with it, the willingness to subordinate individual interests to a greater possibility.
	As the team members grow in their knowledge and trust of one another, they also begin to gain a more accurate picture of the scope of their task, and the team begins to turn towards the task.
	Summing up: the core issue at this stage is trust: 'I believe I can trust the other members of the team'.
The Learning Team	**Willingness** to cooperate is now high, and **skill** in cooperation is beginning to grow, as the group has more experience of working together.
	Having resolved the issues of alignment and trust, the Team is now able to move on to the **task** itself. There are two elements that the Learning Team needs to work through.
	The first is taking ownership of the task they have been given. Although the team may have been given a task when they were formed, they now need to recast that task in their own terms. They need to develop a consensus about what their specific task actually is. If they cannot do that, there are likely to be disagreements about what they are supposed to be doing, and the energies of the group will likely be dissipated in conflict and competition for dominance in setting the direction of the group. Thus, the team needs to fully grasp what the task is and have the ability to articulate it.
	When they can do that, the second element for the Learning Team is to figure out how to accomplish it. Based on the trust they have already built within the Team they can begin to openly discuss the processes and skills which are needed to accomplish the task. Roles are discussed and clarified; and the team asks itself 'How can we cooperate more effectively?' There is more openness, there is greater trust, and people are more willing to help one another. Clearly their **skill** level in cooperation is growing.
	Summing up: the core issues at this stage are ownership of the **task** and agreement about **how** to get the task done.

Table 1 (Continued)

The High-Performance Team	The team is now displaying high *willingness* to cooperate and high *skill* in cooperation. 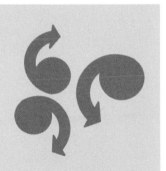
	Having worked through the issues of Alignment, Trust, Task and Process, the Team can now function as a High-Performance Team.
	At this stage, the Team is able to balance the tensions between people and purpose; between individual initiative and collaboration. Everyone is committed to the whole task. There is flexibility and responsiveness. There is a genuine concern about their effectiveness and how they can do better. Group members are in touch with both the task and with one another, and they have learned to balance both task and relationship. People enjoy working together and they are getting the task done, and results can be exceptional!
	The core issue at this stage is commitment to **getting the task accomplished**.

Table 2 Team development – dysfunctional groups

Confused Crowd (high willingness/ low skills)	This group has the best of intentions and a great attitude to working together, but they do not have the skills needed to combine and coordinate their efforts effectively. There is willingness to cooperate, but they just don't have the skills. The problem could stem from inadequate training for the team – or even the make-up of the team (such as missing roles). 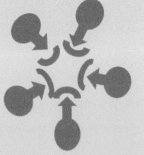
Warring Factions (low willingness/high skills)	This group has skills in cooperation – but they aren't willing to cooperate with one another. The group is characterised by high levels of competition, internal politics or lack of trust. Relationships are so bruised and broken that there is little chance that the individuals will subordinate their interests to the greater needs of the group. In a group like this, it is unlikely that anyone will take the risk of trying to do anything with anybody else; or that there will be any consensus as to who should give any leadership to the group. This group isn't cooperating – and doesn't want to!

(Continued)

Table 2 (Continued)

Unruly Mob (low willingness/low skills)	This group has neither the skills nor the willingness to cooperate. They are made up of individuals who operate independently and who simply want to do it 'my way'! 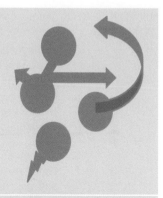
Individual Stars (high skills, but willingness is dependent on their perceived individual interest)	These group members are highly skilled in cooperation, but are in the group for themselves, not for the team. In other words, they don't have the willingness to 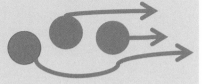 cooperate. It is only when it is to their distinct individual advantage that they use their cooperative skills in a collaborative way. People have high competitive spirits and don't have any trust – and it's almost impossible for a group like this to move up the willingness to cooperate axis.

Appendix 3   My F-words goal sheet

CanChild

My F-words Goal Sheet

f-words
childhood disability

Name: **Today's Date:**

Instructions: Please use this form to **write down one goal for each of the F-words – Function, Family, Fitness, Fun, Friends & Future** and explain **why** this goal is important to you. These can be goals you would like to work on at home, in therapy, in school, and/or in the community. Together let's work on the goals that are meaningful to you!

FUNCTION:

Goal:

Why?!

FAMILY:

Goal:

Why?!

FITNESS:

Goal:

Why?!

FUN:

Goal:

Why?!

FRIENDS:

Goal:

Why?!

FUTURE:

Goal:

Why?!

CanChild

Based on Rosenbaum, P., & Gorter, J.W. (2012). The 'F-words' in Childhood Disability: I swear this is how we should think! *Child: Care, Health and Development*, 38(4). For more information, please visit: www.canchild.ca/f-words

(©CanChild F-words Research Team 2017, adapted from Fuller & Susini Goal Sheet, 2015)

Reprinted with permission from *CanChild 2017*.

Appendix 4   ICF discharge/referral form

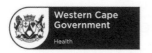
Western Cape Government
Health

RURAL DISTRICT HEALTH SERVICES
ICF version 3.3-2016

INTERPROFESSIONAL PERSON-CENTRED ASSESSMENT AND REFERRAL / DISCHARGE REPORT

1. **Facility** _____

2. **Name:** _____ **Gender** _____

    Folder n: _____ **Date of birth (age)** _____

    Address _____ **Occupation** _____

    _____

    Tel _____

3. **Current health problems / health conditions / health status**
    (Including method of injury, onset, progression, previous treatment, medication)

4. **Medical history** *(e.g. chronic diseases, previous episodes, previous injuries)*

5. **Social history** *(e.g. social determinants of health, grants)*

6.

Outcome level	5: Productive activity	4: Community reintegration	3: Residential integration	2: Physiological maintenance	1: Physiological stability	0: Physiological instability
Initial assessment Date						
Discharge / Referral date						

7. **Special investigations** *(HIV, TB, X-rays, etc.)*

8. **Reason for referral** *(if applicable)*

9. IMPAIRMENT: CHANGES IN BODY FUNCTIONS AND STRUCTURES

Guidance: Use the diagrams below to indicate <u>relevant</u> body impairment and use the space to describe impairment and the actions taken or needed.

CHANGES IN THE FOLLOWING BODY FUNCTIONS?
Mental functions
Sensory functions and pain
Voice and speech functions
Functions of the cardiovascular, haematological, immunological and respiratory systems
Functions of the digestive, metabolic and endocrine systems
Genitourinary and reproductive functions
Neuromusculoskeletal and movement-related functions
Functions of the skin and related structures

CHANGES IN THE FOLLOWING BODY STRUCTURES?
Structures of the nervous system
The eye, ear and related structures
Structures involved in voice and speech
Structures of the cardiovascular, immunological and respiratory systems
Structures related to the digestive, metabolic and endocrine systems
Structures related to the genitourinary and reproductive systems
Structures related to movement
Skin and related structures

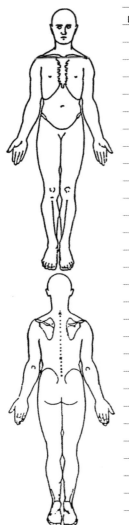

Describe changes in body functions and structures	Actions Needed/Taken

10.   FUNCTIONING

Describe the <u>relevant</u> life areas according to how the person performs during an assessment and/or how the person performs in his/her usual environments (e.g. home, school, community, work).

Domain	Performance	Actions Needed/Taken
Learning & applying knowledge (listening, learning, focusing attention, thinking, making decisions)		
General tasks & demands (undertaking single/multiple tasks, carrying out daily routine, handling stress)		
Communication (receiving and producing messages: spoken, nonverbal, formal sign language, written, devices)		
Mobility (changing and maintaining body position, carrying, objects, walking, moving using transport)		
Self-care (washing oneself, caring for body parts, toileting, dressing, eating, drinking, looking after health)		
Domestic life (acquisition of necessities, place to live, goods, preparing meals, household tasks, assisting others)		
Interpersonal interactions & relationships (formal, family, intimate relationships)		
Major life areas (education, work and employment, economic life)		
Community, social & civic life (community life, recreation, leisure, religion, spirituality, human rights, political)		

11. ENVIRONMENTAL FACTORS

Physical, social and attitudinal factors, external to the individual, that make it easier to function well (facilitators), or if present, are barriers to the way the person lives and conducts his/her life.

Domain	Facilitator (+) Barrier (-)	Actions Needed/Taken
Products & technology (for consumption (food, medication), for use in daily living, mobility, transport, education communication, employment, culture, etc.)		
Physical environment (neighbourhood, housing, sanitation, roads, light, noise, air quality, etc.)		
Support, relationships & attitudes (from immediate/extended family, friends, employer, health professionals, etc.)		
Services, systems and policies (health, housing, transportation, social security, labour, etc.)		

12. Personal factors (positive and negative) influencing health

Background of individual's life and living, which comprise features of the individual that are not part of a health condition or health states. These factors may include gender, race, age, other health conditions, fitness, lifestyle, habits, upbringing, coping styles, ideas, fears, expectations, social background, education, profession, past and current experience (past life events and concurrent events), overall behaviour pattern and character style, individual psychological assets and other characteristics, all or any of which may play a role in disability at any level.

13. PERSON-CENTRED GOAL SETTING AND SHARED DECISION-MAKING

Priority list / unresolved issues	Actions taken/needed

14 Name of Health Professional(s)	Signature	Professional no.	Date and time

Reprinted with permission from Rural District Health Services, Western Cape, South Africa.

Appendix 5 Blank ICF framework

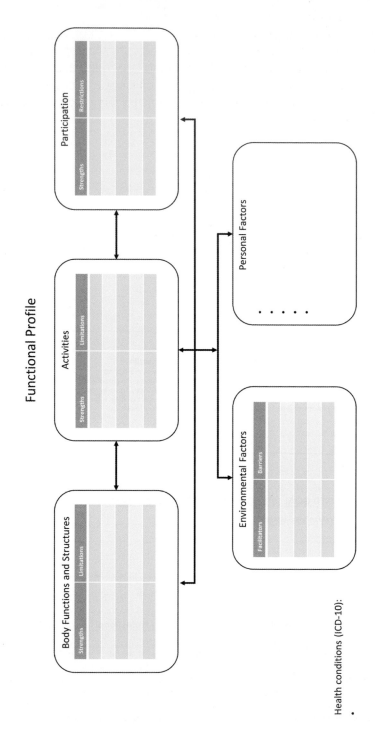

Appendix 6   ICF code sets for children and youth

Code sets for Children and Youth were developed by the German Working Group for the Implementation of the ICF-CY* and registered (#31) at the German Institute for Medical Documentation and Information (DIMDI) (https://dimdi.de/static/de/klassi/icf/projekte/index.htm#beendet). These age-related lists (called checklists in German) are freely available on the websites of some of the participating member associations of the working group:

- German Society for Social Paediatrics and Adolescent Medicine (https://www.dgspj.de/service/icf-cy/)

- Federal Association for People with Physical and Multiple Disabilities (http://bvkm.de/icf-checklisten/)

- German Association for Rehabilitation (https://www.dvfr.de/rehabilitation-und-teilhabe/meldungen-aus-der-reha-landschaft/detail/artikel/anwendung-der-icf-cy-erleichtern/)

An English version of the code sets for children and youth is available to download online at http://www.mackeith.co.uk/shop/icf-a-hands-on-approach-for-clinicians-and-families/

*Composition of the working group: Federal Working Group for Rehabilitation (BAR), Federal Association for People with Cognitive Disabilities (Lebenshilfe), Federal Association for People with Physical and Multiple Disabilities (bvkm), German Society for Social Paediatrics and Adolescent Medicine (DGSPJ), German Association of Occupational Therapists (DVE), German Association for Paediatric Rehabilitation and Prevention (DGPRP), Society for Social Medical Aftercare in Paediatrics (GSNP), Association for Interdisciplinary Early Intervention (VIFF)

Appendix 7   Useful links and additional resources about the ICF

Official WHO ICF website: http://www.who.int/classifications/icf/en/.

ICF Education Website: This website is an online repository of teaching materials about the ICF from around the world. It is maintained by ICF experts, many of them are or were part of the WHO Functioning and Disability Reference Group: http://icfeducation.org.

ICF Research Branch: This website is maintained in cooperation with the German WHO Collaborating Centre (DIMDI) and hosted by the Swiss Paraplegic Centre. It offers materials and courses to different topics of the ICF: https://www.icf-research-branch.org.

F-Words in Childhood Disability Knowledge Hub: This website is hosted by *CanChild* in Canada and provides a collection of resources that have been developed to support knowledge translation and implementation activities related to the ICF: https://www.canchild.ca/en/research-in-practice/f-words-in-childhood-disability/icf-resources.

Needs Assessment Form (NAF) is a downloadable form for prescribing assistive devices based on the ICF used in Germany and available in English: https://www.rehakind.de/m.php?sid=60.

Index

NOTES: Figures, tables & boxes are denoted by a lower case italic in the page reference (*f*, *t* and *b* respectively). The "International Classification of Functionality, Disability and Health" is abbreviated to ICF, and "Patient Reported Outcome Measures" to PROMs, in subheadings throughout.

Other titles from Mac Keith Press   www.mackeith.co.uk

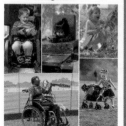

Children and Youth with Complex Cerebral Palsy: Care and Management
Laurie J. Glader and Richard D. Stevenson (Editors)

A practical guide from Mac Keith Press
2019 ▪ 404pp ▪ softback ▪ 978-1-909962-98-9

This is the first practical guide to explore management of the many medical comorbidities that children with complex CP face, including orthopaedics, mobility needs, cognition and sensory impairment, difficult behaviours, respiratory complications and nutrition, amongst others. Uniquely, contributors include children and parents, providing applied wisdom for family-centred care. Clinical Care Tools are provided to help guide clinicians and include a Medical Review Supplement, Equipment and Services Checklist and an ICF-Based Care: Goals and Management Form.

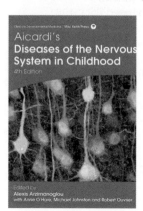

Aicardi's Diseases of the Nervous System in Childhood, 4th Edition
Alexis Arzimanoglou, Anne O'Hare, Michael V Johnston and Robert Ouvrier (Editors)

Clinics in Developmental Medicine
2018 ▪ 1524pp ▪ softback ▪ 978-1-909962-80-4

This fourth edition retains the patient-focussed, clinical approach of its predecessors. The international team of editors and contributors has honoured the request of the late Jean Aicardi, that his book remain 'resolutely clinical', which distinguishes *Diseases of the Nervous System in Childhood* from other texts in the field. New edition completely updated and revised and now in full colour.

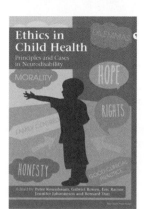

Ethics in Child Health: Principles and Cases in Neurodisability
Peter L. Rosenbaum, Gabriel M. Ronen, Eric Racine, Jennifer Johannesen and Bernard Dan (Editors)

A practical guide from Mac Keith Press
2016 ▪ 396pp ▪ softback ▪ 978-1-909962-63-7

This book explores the ethical dimensions of issues that have either been ignored or not recognised. Each chapter is built around an illustrative scenario and discusses how ethical principles can be utilised to inform decision-making. 'Themes for Discussion' at the end of each chapter will help professionals and policy makers put practical ethical thinking at the heart of care.

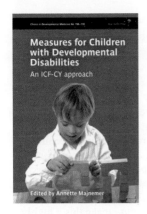

Measures for Children with Developmental Disabilities: An ICF-CY approach
Annette Majnemer (Editor)

Clinics in Developmental Medicine No 194-195
2012 ▪ 552pp ▪ hardback ▪ 978-1-908316-45-5

This title presents and reviews outcome measures across a wide range of attributes that are applicable to children and adolescents with developmental disabilities. It uses the children and youth version of the International Classification of Functioning, Disability and Health (ICF-CY) as a framework for organizing the various measures into sections and chapters. Each chapter coincides with domains within the WHO framework of Body Functions, Activities and Participation, and Personal and Environmental Factors.

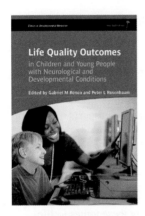

Life Quality Outcomes in Children and Young People with Neurological and Developmental Conditions
Gabriel M. Ronen and Peter L. Rosenbaum (Editors)

Clinics in Developmental Medicine
2013 ▪ 394pp ▪ hardback ▪ 978-1-908316-58-5

Healthcare professionals need to understand their patients' views of their condition and its effects on their health and well-being. This book builds on the World Health Organization's concepts of 'health', 'functioning' and 'quality of life' for young people with neurodisabilities: it emphasises the importance of engaging with patients in the identification of both treatment goals and their evaluation. Uniquely, it enables healthcare professionals to find critically reviewed outcomes-related information.

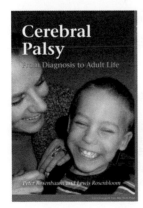

Cerebral Palsy: From Diagnosis to Adult Life
Peter L. Rosenbaum and Lewis Rosenbloom (Editors)

A practical guide from Mac Keith Press
2012 ▪ 224pp ▪ softback ▪ 978-1-908316-50-9

This book has been designed to provide readers with an understanding of cerebral palsy as a developmental as well as a neurological condition. It details the nature of cerebral palsy, its causes and its clinical manifestations. Using clear, accessible language (supported by an extensive glossary) the authors have blended current science with metaphor to explain the biomedical underpinnings of cerebral palsy.

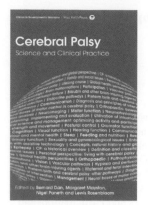

Cerebral Palsy: Science and Clinical Practice
Bernard Dan, Margaret Mayston, Nigel Paneth and Lewis Rosenbloom (Editors)

Clinics in Developmental Medicine
2015 ▪ 648pp ▪ hardback ▪ 978-1-909962-38-5

This landmark title considers all aspects of cerebral palsy from the causes to clinical problems and their implications for individuals. An international team of experts present a wide range of person-centred assessment approaches, including clinical evaluation, measurement scales, neuroimaging and gait analysis. The perspective of the book spans the lifelong course of cerebral palsy, taking into account worldwide differences in socio-economic and cultural factors. Full integrated colour, with extensive cross-referencing make this a highly attractive and useful reference.

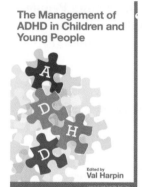

The Management of ADHD in Children and Young People
Val Harpin (Editor)

A practical guide from Mac Keith Press
2017 ▪ 292pp ▪ softback ▪ 978-1-909962-72-9

This book is an accessible and practical guide on all aspects of assessment of children and young people with Attention Deficit Hyperactivity Disorder (ADHD) and how they can be managed successfully. The multi-professional team of authors discusses referral, assessment and diagnosis, psychological management, pharmacological management, and co-existing conditions, as well as ADHD in the school setting. New research on girls with ADHD is also featured. Case scenarios are included that bring these topics to life.

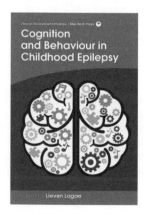

Cognition and Behaviour in Childhood Epilepsy
Lieven Lagae (Editor)

Clinics in Developmental Medicine
2017 ▪ 186pp ▪ hardback ▪ 978-1-909962-87-3

For many parents, cognitive and behavioral comorbidities, such as ADHD, autism and intellectual disability, are the real burden of childhood epilepsy. This title offers concrete guidance and treatment strategies for childhood epilepsy in general, and for the comorbidities associated with each epilepsy syndrome and their pathophysiology. The book is written by experts in the field with an important clinical experience, while chapters by clinical neuropsychologists provide a strong theoretical background.

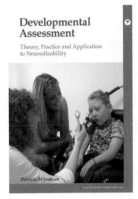

Developmental Assessment: Theory, Practice and Application to Neurodisability
Patricia M. Sonksen

A practical guide from Mac Keith Press
2016 ▪ 384pp ▪ softback ▪ 978-1-909962-56-9

This handbook presents a new approach to assessing development in preschool children that can be applied across the developmental spectrum. The reader is taught how to confirm whether development is typical, and if it is not, is signposted to the likely nature and severity of the impairments with a plan of action. The author uses numerous case vignettes from her 40 years' experience to bring to life her approach with clear summary key points and helpful illustrations.

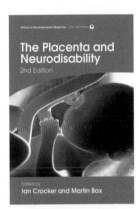

The Placenta and Neurodisability, 2nd Edition
Ian Crocker and Martin Bax (Editors)

Clinics in Developmental Medicine
2015 ▪ 176pp ▪ hardback ▪ 978-1-909962-53-8

This comprehensive and authoritative book discusses the critical role of the utero-placenta in neurodisability, both at term and preterm. It examines aspects of fetal compromise and possible cerebro-protective interventions, recent evidence on fetal growth and mental illness, as well as cerebro-therapeutics. Throughout the book, information from the basic sciences is placed within the clinical context.

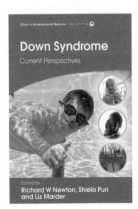

Down Syndrome: Current Perspectives
Richard W. Newton, Shiela Puri and Liz Marder (Editors)

Clinics in Developmental Medicine
2015 ▪ 320pp ▪ hardback ▪ 978-1-909962-47-7

Down syndrome remains the most common recognisable form of intellectual disability. The challenge for doctors today is how to capture the rapidly expanding body of scientific knowledge and devise models of care to meet the needs of individuals and their families. *Down Syndrome: Current Perspectives* provides doctors and other health professionals with the information they need to address the challenges that can present in the management of this syndrome.